Contents

Letter from the editor	2
Explore your options	4, 5
Diana Award	6
The Alternatives to University Section	7 to 10
Degree apprenticeships / Law	11
Jones Day	12, 13
The University Section	
Why go to uni?	16, 17
How to choose course & uni	18, 19
University league tables	20
The best online resources	22
Uni open days	24
Applying to Oxford or Cambridge	26 to 29
Applying through UCAS	30 to 33
How to handle A-Level results day	34 to 37
Personal statement masterclass	38 to 47
Example personal statement	48
Enrichment	49
Boost your personal statement	50, 51
University interviews	52 to 55
University of Kent	14
University of Manchester	21
Imperial College, London	23
UCL	25
Student finance	56
A note from Martin Lewis	57
Budgeting by Save the Student	58, 59
Freshers' Week	60, 61
Making the most of your time at uni	62
Changing your course / dropping out	63
Working for your uni	64, 65
Debate Mate	66, 67
Generate Talks	78
Studying abroad	68, 69
USA	70
Australia & New Zealand	71
Europe	72
My experience	73
Harvard University	74, 75
Gap years	76, 77
Career Profiles Section	
What are you going to do with your life?	80, 81
What Career Live?	82, 83
Healthcare	84
Medical applicants	85
Getting into medical school	86, 87
Alternatives routes into medicine	88
My experience	89
Finance	90
EY	91
KPMG	92, 93
ICAEW	94, 95
Law	96, 98, 100
Barristers	102, 103
Gowling WLG	97
Stephenson Harwood	99
Herbert Smith Freehills	101
Intellectual property	103 to 106
Original Steps career profiles	107 to 116
The Job Crowd	118
The Job Applications Section	
Work experience	120, 121
Employability skills	122, 123
CV writing masterclass	124, 126
Using LinkedIn	127
The covering letter	128, 129
Application forms	130
Types of questions	131, 132
Assessment days	133
Job interviews	134, 135

Explore your options

It can be hard to figure out where to start when thinking about the future. Follow the decision tree below to give you an idea of what next steps you could take. We always recommend exploring all your options before making a final decision, so approach this with an open mind. If you decide to take a gap year inbetween, you'll still need to plan ahead whichever path you follow.

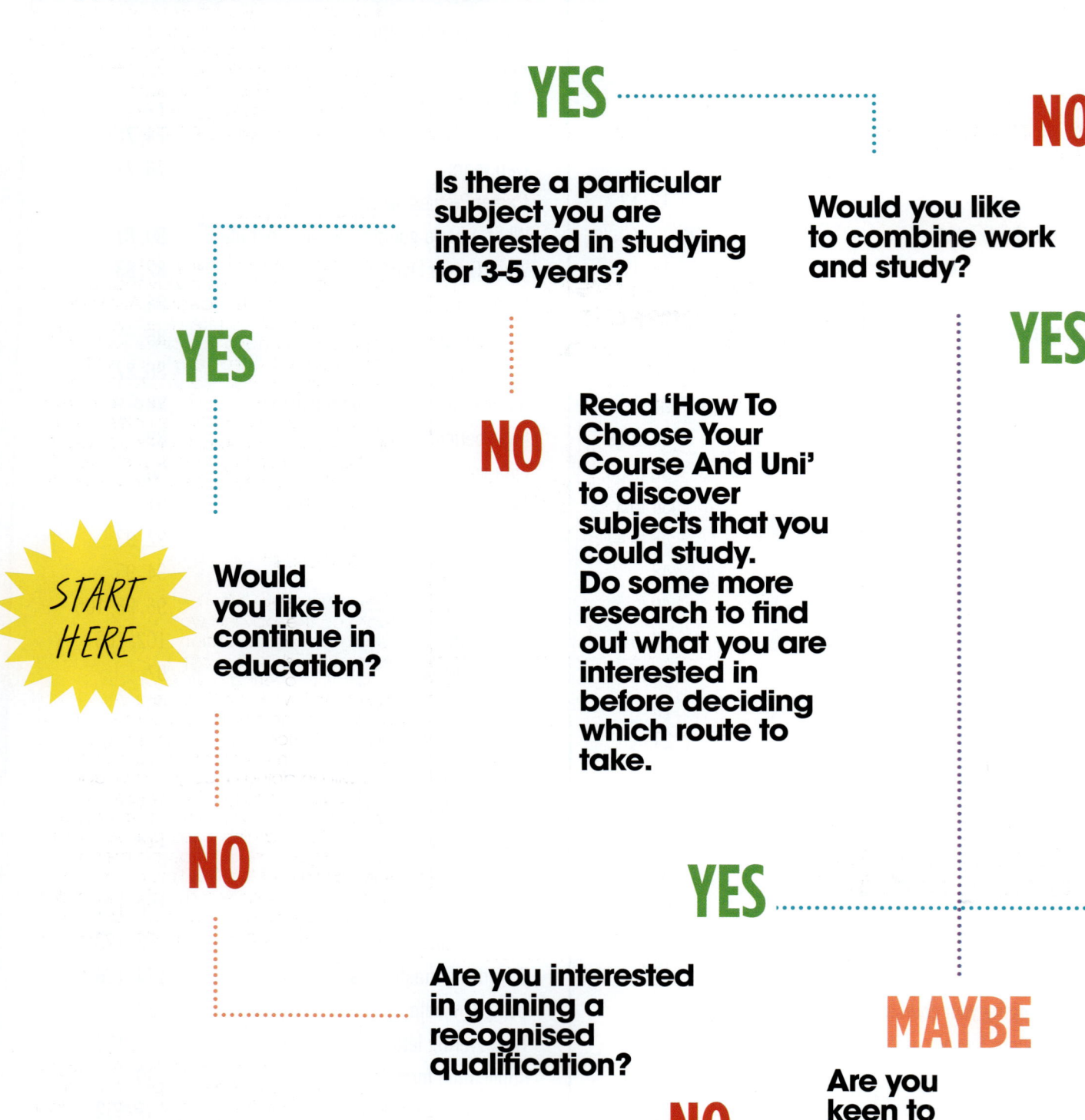

START HERE

Would you like to continue in education?

- **YES** → **Is there a particular subject you are interested in studying for 3-5 years?**
  - **YES** → **Would you like to combine work and study?**
    - **NO**
    - **YES**
  - **NO** → Read 'How To Choose Your Course And Uni' to discover subjects that you could study. Do some more research to find out what you are interested in before deciding which route to take.

- **NO** → **Are you interested in gaining a recognised qualification?**
  - **YES**
  - **MAYBE** → **Are you keen to start earning a full time wage?**
    - **NO**
    - **YES**

Reproduction in whole or in part without written permission is strictly prohibited. © 2018 Pure Potential Ltd.

Do you want to experience university life?

YES ········· EDUCATION

NO

Would you prefer to be based in a workplace or an educational institution?

········· WORKPLACE

READING

Do you learn best by reading or doing?

········· DOING

NO

DEGREE

Studying towards a degree at university has many benefits. It means you can engross yourself in a subject that really interests you. Alongside the academic side of university, you will also make lots of new friends, have the opportunity to take up new hobbies and experience living away from home. Finding part time work alongside your studies or during the holidays will enable you to gain skills and earn some extra money. Read through the university section of APPLY, for information on how to research universities, choosing a subject and the whole UCAS application process.

DEGREE APPRENTICESHIP

A degree apprenticeship (aka sponsored degree) is a way that you can work towards a degree AND be employed at the same time, meaning generally you have your fees paid and earn money along the way, as well as developing contacts and skills that a degree alone won't offer you. Your time will usually be split between attending university and working for the company that are sponsoring your degree. Read more about these in the alternatives to uni section.

APPRENTICESHIP

Apprenticeships offer a great way to learn on the job and work towards a recognised qualification. Apprenticeships are offered in 170 industries covering over 1,500 job roles, including law! Even if you answered you didn't want to combine work and study, an apprenticeship isn't like going to college or university. As an apprentice you will be doing a real job in a real workplace – and getting paid for it. Learning on an apprenticeship will be different to learning at school, so if you didn't enjoy school it doesn't mean education isn't for you! Having a nationally recognised qualification will stand you in good stead for your future career. Read more in the alternatives to uni section.

WORK

For some people going into work straight away has many benefits. Spend some time whilst at sixth form or college to gain some work experience, networks and employability skills. There are lots of great opportunities out there for school leavers so make sure you read the school leaver section. Remember you can return to education at any age and there are many options for studying part time alongside work if you change your mind about education in the future.

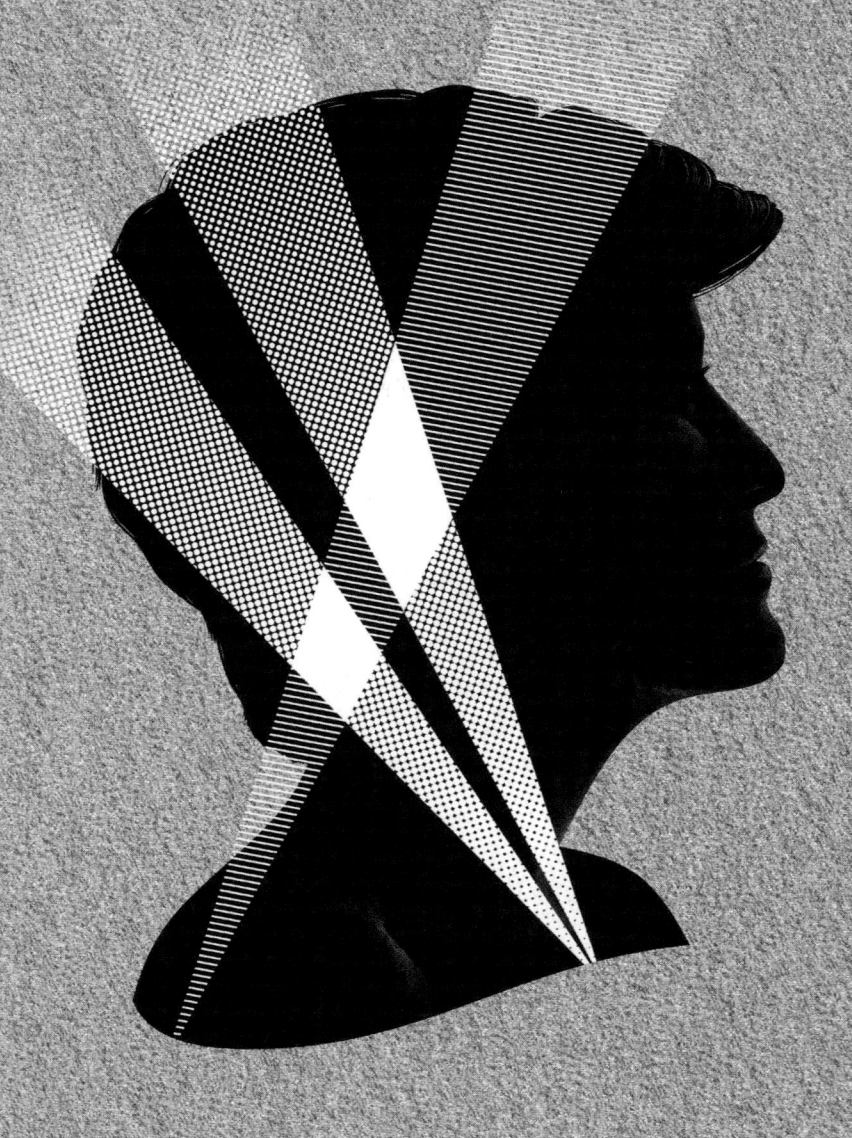

NOMINATE FOR_THE DIANA AWARD

DO YOU KNOW A YOUNG PERSON WHO IS SELFLESSLY TRANSFORMING THE LIVES OF OTHERS? A YOUNG HUMANITARIAN, DEDICATED VOLUNTEER, PASSIONATE CAMPAIGNER OR DETERMINED FUNDRAISER?

2018 NOMINATIONS NOW OPEN
diana-award.org.uk/nominate

APPLY

THE
ALTERNATIVES
TO
UNI
SECTION

2018

SCHOOL LEAVER PROGRAMMES

School leaver programes offer you the chance to earn a competitive salary, gain qualifications and get real-life commercial experience. We think a good place to start is by dispelling some common myths:

MYTH 1 – "School leaver programmes aren't well-respected"

There are over 300 leading employers who offer competitive programmes with many more each year. With recent changes in higher education, employers predicted a decline in the number of students applying to university and decided to offer an attractive alternative for smart, ambitious students. The 'rise of the school leaver programme' has caused a shift in employment, and companies are quickly realising the talent, enthusiasm and fresh ideas younger students can bring to their organisations. They are investing time and money into hiring, training and developing their school leaver workforce – this definitely would not be happening if employers did not consider school leaver programmes a well-respected route. This shift in focus is causing a stir amongst students, parents and teachers – there are more students than ever before opting to go down the school leaver route and an increasing number of teachers and parents are supporting this move too.

MYTH 2 – "A university degree is your passport to employment whereas a school leaver programme can only get you so far"

There was once a time when you could waltz out of university with a degree and land yourself a first-class job. Unfortunately, times have changed, and with thousands of graduates entering the job market each year, students are now required to go the extra mile (or two) to get a job when they leave university, and there are many who are still unemployed. The majority of school leaver employers offer reputable professional qualifications as part of their programme (including some employers who run degree apprenticeships). These professional qualifications are widely recognised and can be your passport for working not just in the UK but around the globe! In some cases, you could even complete your qualification faster than if you were to go down the university route. You can also make excellent professional connections which will be valuable further down the line if you decided to move jobs.

MYTH 3 – "School leavers aren't paid well"

The vast majority of school leaver providers pay their school leavers a competitive salary and they cover the cost of all training and any qualifications they gain, which can be very expensive! Salaries usually increase as you progress through the programme and take on more responsibilities which means you will have more money to spend or to put towards buying your first home.

MYTH 4 – "School leavers miss out on the social life that university provides"

Without doubt, university is a lot of fun – you spend three years having a great time, making friends and develop a lot of life skills. Employers recognise that students are giving up three years of socialising and more, which is why they often have a dedicated team that looks after social activities for new starters. They will organise away days, team building retreats and regular social events to give you a chance to meet new people, make friends and build that all-important social network.

It's important that you think carefully about what you want to do after sixth form. If you're not sure whether a school leaver programme would be a good fit for you, considering the pros and cons might help:

PROS

- Gain a professional qualification
- Earn a competitive salary
- Get first-hand, real experience with professionals
- No student debt
- There is less competition for places at school-leaver level than graduate level
- You can be financially independent – and not reliant on loans
- Many companies offer the chance to try different areas of the business which can help you find out what you enjoy
- You will receive extensive training by leading professionals in a structured programme
- Some companies offer students the chance to study part-time at university and gain a degree alongside working

CONS

- You'll have to make a decision about where to begin your career sooner than some of your peers
- You might feel worried you're missing out on some of the experiences that your friends who go to university are having

WHAT ARE THE OPTIONS?

The difference between the following programmes and just getting an ordinary job is that schools leavers programmes offer a training schedule, qualifications or progression infrastructure of some sort. These programmes are a launch pad into an advanced career level, which is why they are so sought after! Here is a brief guide to each type, but check each company's specifications because they vary enormously.

SCHOOL LEAVER PROGRAMMES

A school leaver programme is a fixed-term, paid job available to students after sixth form which provides an intensive, structured training programme and in some cases formal professional qualifications.

APPRENTICESHIPS

An apprenticeship is usually referred to as a job in a vocational industry where young people can train while they earn money from the age of 16 in careers as diverse as nursing, engineering, finance, and carpentry. Confusingly, some professional school leaver programmes are also known as apprenticeships.

HIGHER APPRENTICESHIPS

These are paid apprenticeships that give you the chance to progress academically to degree level (such as NVQ levels 4&5, Foundation Degrees, HNCs or HNDs) through practical work experience.

DEGREE APPRENTICESHIP

As the name suggests you will work towards a degree as part of the programme, normally whilst working as a permanent employee for the organisation and normally with your fees paid for!

APPRENTICESHIPS AND HIGHER APPRENTICESHIPS

Work with some of the most exciting and innovative companies across the country straight out of sixth form.

What is the difference between an Apprenticeship and a Higher Apprenticeship?

There are various levels of apprenticeship you can undertake depending on the skills and qualifications that you leave school or college with a Higher Apprenticeship. This is a nationally accredited work-based programme designed to meet employers' needs at higher skill levels and include qualifications at a level equivalent to higher education. There are three levels of apprenticeship:

- Intermediate Apprenticeships, which are equivalent to five good GCSEs

- Advanced Level Apprenticeships, which are equivalent to two A-levels

- Higher Apprenticeships, which can lead to a HND, HNC or foundation degree

You should note that...

Higher levels might require more qualifications: for example, some Higher Apprenticeships require you to have A-levels.

Apprenticeships in some areas are only available at particular levels. For example, Emergency Care is only available as an Intermediate Apprenticeship.

Your apprenticeship may last longer at a higher level, although this can vary. There are fewer apprenticeships available at Higher level than at the other levels.

A Higher Apprenticeship can lead to a professional qualification, such as a Certificate in Finance, Accounting and Business (CFAB).

Will I earn money?

All apprentices earn a salary and will work for at least 30 hours per week.

How long do apprenticeships take?

An apprenticeship takes between one and five years to complete, depending upon the level of apprenticeship and the industry sector.

What will an apprenticeship be like day-to-day?

Most of the training is delivered in the workplace, so you will learn the skills you need to do the job well. The rest is given by a training organisation, either at the workplace, off-site (perhaps at college) or via online courses. The training is specifically tailored to ensure you develop the skills the employer wants, giving apprentices a real advantage in the workplace.

"I knew that going to university wasn't the right decision for me. I didn't want to spend the next couple of years learning in a school-like environment without being able to apply my skills to the working world."

WHY THEY ARE A RESPECTABLE ALTERNATIVE

Helpful discussion points to talk through with anyone sceptical about school leaver programmes

You are bright, talented and full of ambition. No doubt your teacher, parent or carer you will want to support you as you make crucial decisions for your future but the school leaver market is relatively new and they may have concerns or hesitations if you show an interest in this path.

Whatever you go on to do it is important that your family and teachers are involved in the decision-making process and are able to offer informed guidance.

Talking is the best way to build an understanding of the career paths you're thinking about - here are some ideas:

- **HAVE YOU CONSIDERED THE PROS AND CONS FOR SCHOOL LEAVER PROGRAMMES AND UNIVERSITY?**
- **HAVE YOU LOOKED INTO THE APPLICATION PROCESS? WHAT IS INVOLVED? WHAT ARE YOUR LONG TERM CAREER PROSPECTS?**
- **EXPLAIN WHY YOU ARE THINKING ABOUT APPLYING FOR A SCHOOL LEAVER PROGRAMME**
- **HAVE YOU DONE LOTS OF RESEARCH ON THE TYPE OF PROGRAMMES OUT THERE?**
- **HOW DOES YOUR CAREER PATH COMPARE TO THE UNIVERSITY ROUTE?**
- **WILL YOU APPLY TO UNI TO KEEP YOUR OPTIONS OPEN?**
- **WHICH PARTICULAR PROGRAMMES OR COMPANIES HAVE YOU RESEARCHED?**
- **HAVE YOU SPOKEN TO ANY SCHOOL LEAVERS? WHAT DO THEY THINK OF THEIR CHOSEN PATH?**

USEFUL RESOURCES

When making a big decision, like what to do after leaving sixth form, it's a good idea to be as informed as possible. We've put together a list of all the best that's out there on the web to check out when considering your options:

www.purepotential.org
You can register your e-mail and receive alerts about events and opportunities from us and our partner employers that will help give you greater insight into your future options.

www.apprenticeships.gov.uk
Has lots of information for both students and their teachers, parents or carers about all of the different apprenticeships on offer and how to access them.

www.schoolleavers.milkround.com
Has live vacancies and advice and information on most school leaver programmes with major employers.

www.allaboutschoolleavers.co.uk
Pretty much does what it says on the tin! All About School Leavers has lots of information about all of the different options out there as well as advice about hot to make a great application.

www.ratemyapprenticeship.co.uk
Want to know what previous school leavers have thought about their experiences with employers? This site enables people to review their school leaver programme (like you would a restaurant or hotel) which can be really helpful when deciding which schemes you might want to apply for. It also has a brilliant 'advice hub' with articles, discussions and news about what's going on in the world of school leavers.

www.studentladder.co.uk
Has a comprehensive school leaver section with different opportunities split out by industry, making it easy to find schemes you might be interested in.

www.thebigchoice.com
Answers the big questions about school leaver programmes in different sectors, such as 'what's it all about?', 'where can I work? And 'how much can I earn?'. Also features lots of school leaver job opportunities to apply for.

DEGREE APPRENTICESHIPS

Degree apprenticeships (AKA sponsored degrees) are becoming increasingly popular and it's no wonder why – they allow you to go to university and get a degree whilst having your tuition fees paid for and earning a salary. What's not to like?

What is a degree apprenticeship programme?

A degree apprenticeship acts as an alternative for those who wish to gain a degree qualification but do not necessarily want to attend higher education full time.

Degree apprenticeships are made up of both employment and study. Your time will generally be split between attending university and working for the company that are sponsoring your degree – meaning you gain both a qualification and valuable work experience.

Are all programmes the same?

Degree apprenticeship programmes can really vary. Depending on the programme, you might attend university in person or undertake a distance learning course remotely from home or your employer's office. For those courses where you will physically attend university, the amount of time you spend there will differ for each course.

For some you may do one or two days of the week at university and be in the office the rest of the time. For others, you might attend university on a full-time basis, and just spend holidays working for the company.

Some programmes will offer only a specific degree from a specific institution whereas others provide some choice in where you study and what qualification you work towards. There are also slightly different forms of sponsorship that act more like a scholarship, with universities sponsoring students irrespective of their course or university. Students might undertake work placements or graduate schemes with the employer in return.

What are the benefits?

There are plenty!

- Getting to study towards and gain a degree, an internationally recognised qualification which you can refer to throughout the rest of your working life
- Having your university fees paid for/contributed to and potentially avoiding thousands of pounds worth of student debt
- Earning a salary whilst you study
- Access to work experience with a professional employer and an opportunity to develop valuable skills
- The likelihood that once your sponsored degree programme reaches its conclusion, you'll be offered a graduate position with the company.

Any downsides?

By choosing to work whilst studying you might feel like you're missing out on the full uni experience. Also, it's likely that your employer will only sponsor a specific course at a specific university so you might not get much choice in what you study. These degree programmes are definitely suited to those of you who have a clear idea of what you want to do as a career. If you're unsure at this stage then a more generic degree course may be right for you.

Where can I find out more about degree apprenticeships?

Big companies are increasingly offering degree apprenticeships. If you think you might be interested in sponsored degrees then start researching online. Think about the industries and employers you would like to work for in the future and then go and see if they offer a degree apprenticeship.

Many of Pure Potential's partners offer degree apprenticeship programmes so it's worth registering at www.purepotential.org for events where you can meet a sponsored degree programme provider.

LEGAL APPRENTICESHIPS

(with thanks to Get My First Job)

It is no longer essential to go to university to gain a qualification in law!

The new Legal Services Apprenticeship Programmes offer you the opportunity to study law as you gain real experience and you'll be getting paid!

Law apprenticeships offer a great progression route taking you from a level 2 intermediate qualification all the way up to a level 7 masters degree to become a qualified solicitor.

Law Apprenticeship Programmes

You could be working in a variety of roles depending on the sector your employer covers and the level of your apprenticeship. The current legal apprenticeships available are:

Legal Advice
– Level 2 Intermediate & Level 3 Advanced

Legal Services
– Level 3 Advanced & Level 4 Higher Paralegal
– Level 3 Advanced

Chartered Legal Executive
– Level 6 Higher

Solicitor
– Level 7 Masters Degree

Legal Advice:

Legal advisers are on hand to offer independent advice and guidance to members of the public on their rights, entitlements and responsibilities under the law.

Legal Services & Paralegal:

Paralegals or Legal Assistants have some legal training but are not qualified as either a Lawyer, Barrister or Solicitor and form an important part of the legal team. They normally work for, or under supervision of a qualified legal practitioner to progress case files or specific parts of the legal process.

MY EXPERIENCE

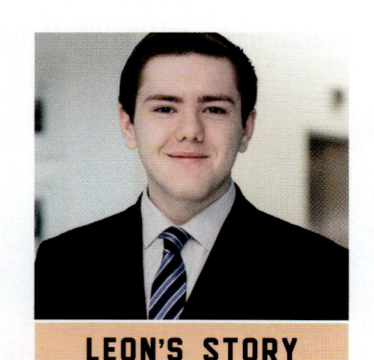

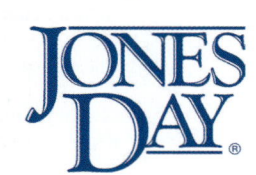

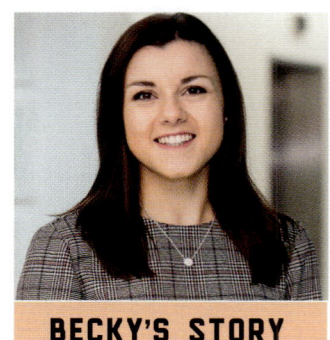

LEON'S STORY

"I decided to pursue an apprenticeship straight after BTEC at college rather than enter higher education as I felt that actual corporate experience could be just as valuable to me as a university qualification. I had chosen BTECs rather than conventional A-Levels because I found that completing a wide range of assignments and case studies over time suited me better than studying for one-off exams and I felt an apprenticeship would replicate that style of learning in the work place.

This particular apprenticeship at Jones Day combines study at BPP University one day a week with 4 days a week working at Jones Day and provides full support towards both a Paralegal Qualification (first two years) and a Solicitor Qualification (with law degree) (following 5 years). All study costs for the 7 year apprenticeship period are covered and I am paid a salary as well. Now in my second year of the Paralegal Apprenticeship, I hope to advance to the Solicitor Apprenticeship, incorporating an LLB Law degree, at the end of this year. So I have been able to move forward academically and at work without the worries that come with student debt.

The best thing about the Jones Day apprenticeship is the diverse range of work I do. As Jones Day do not have a rotational or "seat" training system, I get the opportunity to work with numerous departments at the same time. I didn't want to spend my entire apprenticeship with one team as I felt that would limit my development and my choice of specialization. Jones Day offer their apprentices the chance to try every sector which means I gain a greater knowledge of several different areas of law and can choose which area suits me.

I am one of the first generation of apprentices at Jones Day. My greatest surprise has been how quickly I have progressed in the year I have been here. I have exceeded my own expectations and developed skills such as time-management, attention to detail and problem solving. When applying for the apprenticeship, I admit I found the size of the Firm and the work it does fairly daunting. But I quickly learned that everyone is incredibly friendly and wants me to succeed and feel comfortable here."

BECKY'S STORY

"I chose this legal apprenticeship over my offer of a place at university because it would provide me with the opportunity to gain valuable skills in the workplace, whilst also studying for a law degree and (hopefully!) qualifying as a solicitor. Jones Day's full, seven year apprenticeship programme may seem like a long time at first, but it will actually take me the same amount of time to qualify as a solicitor as if I'd studied the non-law degree I had a place for at university. The apprenticeship has given me hands-on experience and a practical way of learning what a lawyer really does.

A lot of my friends are at university and admittedly are all having a great time. However, a lot of them have said they are envious that I am gaining workplace experience whilst they are struggling to find work placements, internships and jobs. I'm also earning a good salary!

The best thing about the Jones Day apprenticeship is the varied work I do. As Jones Day do not require me to sit with a specific team in a specific "seat", I am able to get involved in work from all of the different departments at the same time. I have also been surprised by the type of work I can do. I thought being one of the most junior in the office I would be doing solely administrative tasks. In reality I complete substantive work including legal research and drafting letters. I have even attended a trial. From an early stage I have been actively involved in very high value cases and deals which is an exciting advantage of working at a large, global firm like Jones Day.

Now in my second year of the 2 year Paralegal Apprenticeship, I see my role in the Firm expanding. I hope to continue to improve my knowledge of the law in a practical context by continuing my involvement in substantive work and seeing cases and deals through from start to finish. My aim is to move onto the 5 year Solicitor Apprenticeship, incorporating an LLB Law degree, next year."

JONES DAY | One Firm Worldwide℠

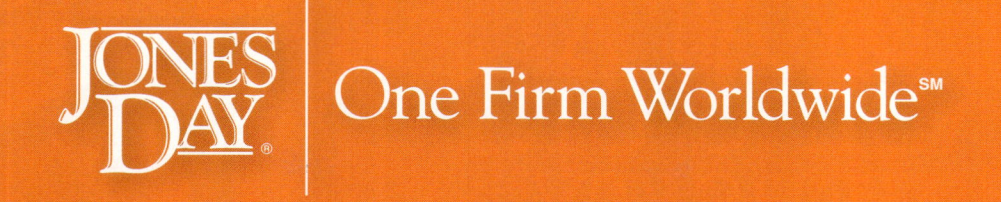

Earn & Learn as a Legal Apprentice

Start as a two-year Paralegal Apprentice
Graduate to a five-year Solicitor Apprentice
Qualify as a solicitor after seven years

Work across teams & practice areas
Achieve a law degree without the fees

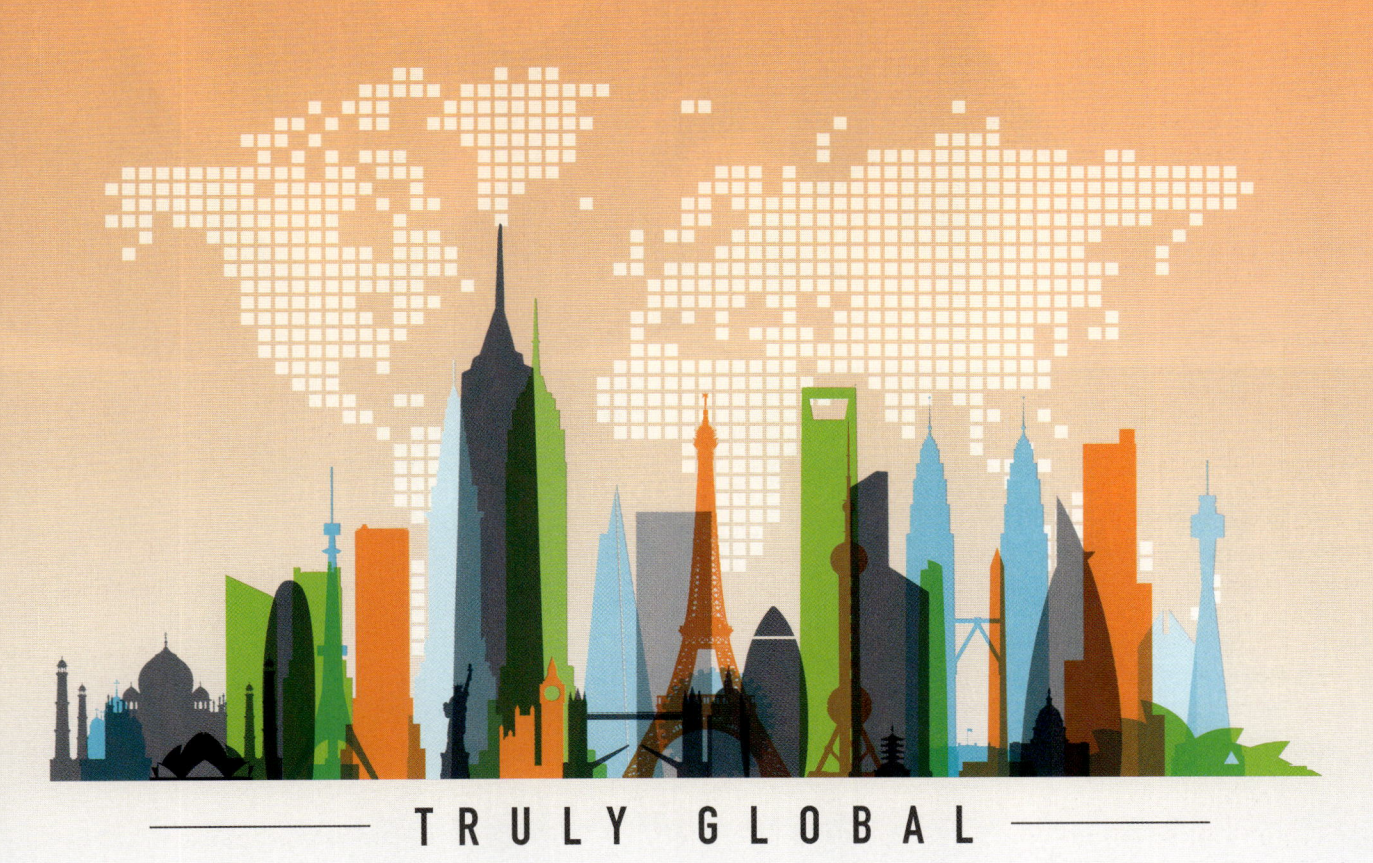

TRULY GLOBAL

Litigation Powerhouse • Collaborative Not Competitive Culture • No Law Firm Does More M&A

Applications open 15.12.17 – 21.01.18
Apply via GetMyFirstJob.com

For more information visit www.jonesdaylondon.com

STUDY AT A LEADING UK UNIVERSITY

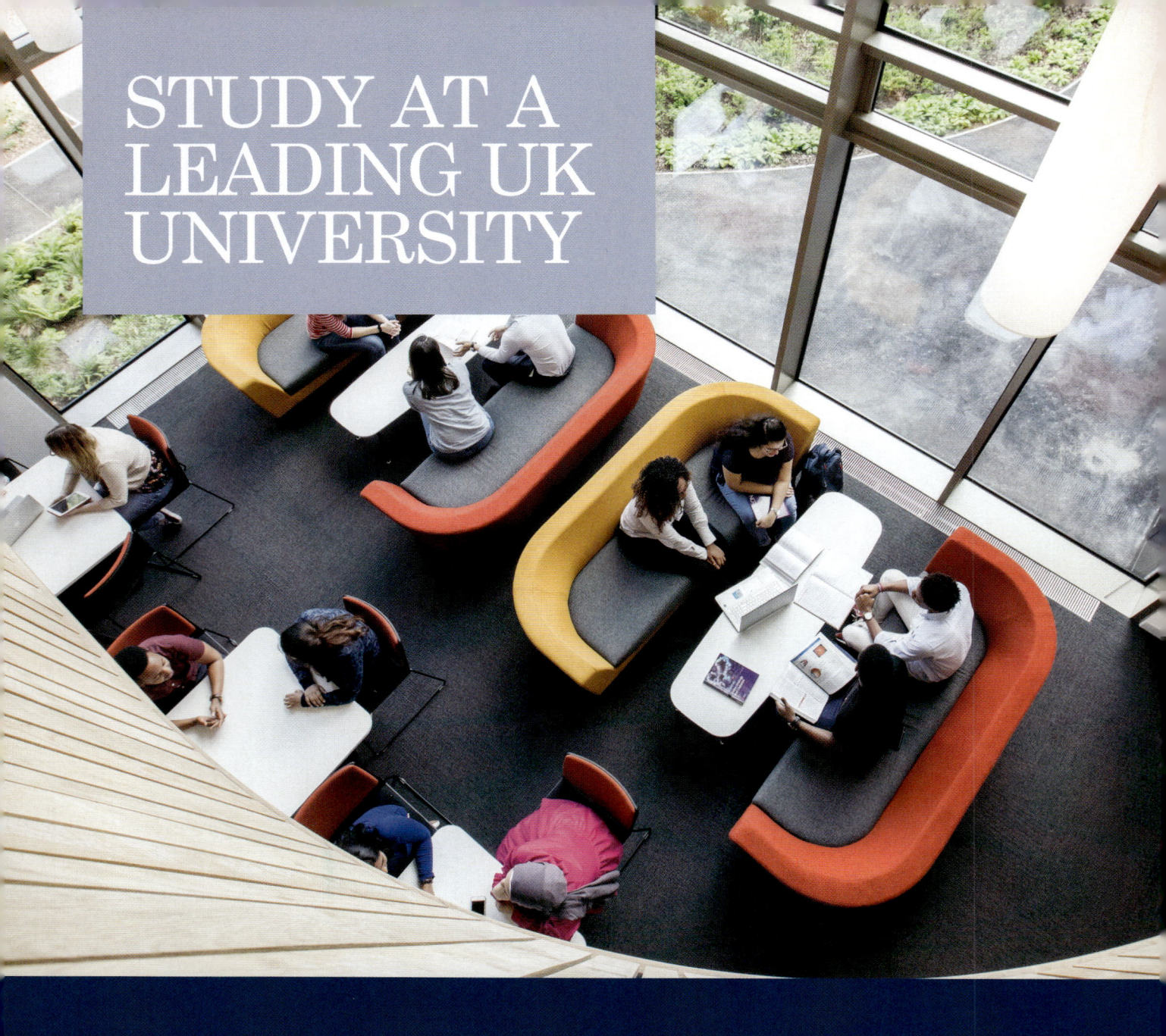

Kent offers academic excellence, inspirational teaching and a superb student experience.

- £2,000 scholarship to all students achieving AAA (A level) / DDD (BTEC) / IB35*
- Ranked 22nd in the *Guardian University Guide 2018*
- 96% of Kent's students who graduated in 2016 found a job or a study opportunity within 6 months
- Our Canterbury campus has fantastic facilities including a nightclub, cinema and sports centre all set in 300 acres of parkland.
- Our Medway campus has high-tech facilities, a great riverside location and is only 30 miles from London.

To find out more come along to an Open Day
www.kent.ac.uk/opendays

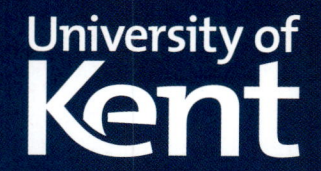

* see website for specified equivalents and conditions

TEF Gold Teaching Excellence Framework

University of Kent

APPLY

The University Section

2018

Why go to university?

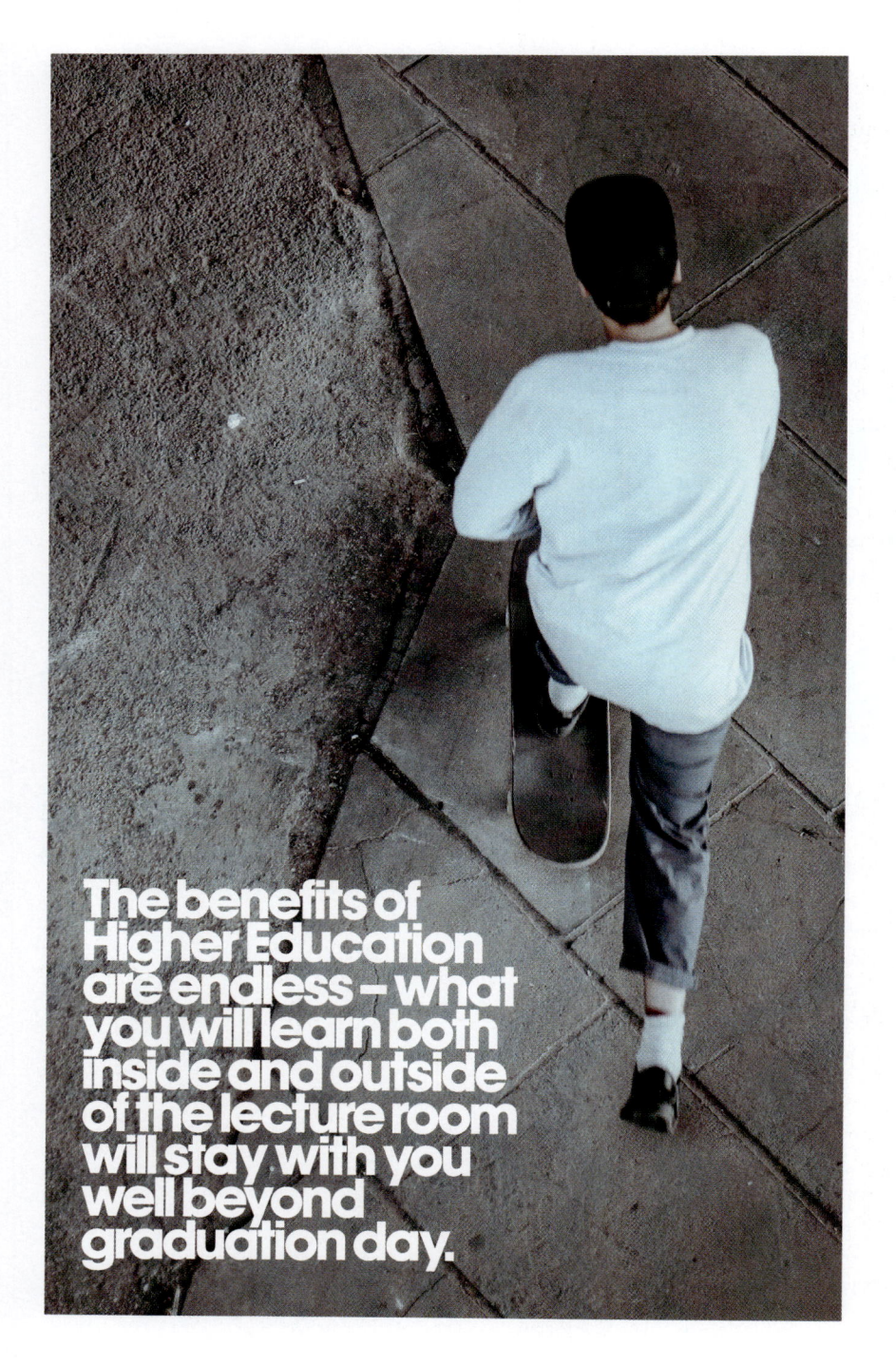

With tuition fees of up to £9,250 a year, many students will be wondering whether it's worthwhile going to university. Not everyone's dream will involve higher education, and nor should it. Many top athletes, musicians, tech pros and business gurus choose not to go to university, but go on to achieve great things.

There is nothing wrong with opting out of the university route, but you should carefully consider all your options before you make a decision – you can read about the alternatives to university later on.

In many areas of life however, a university degree is still an essential route. If you want to become a doctor, dentist or vet, develop new treatments, delve into histroy and the arts, understand the sciences and our environment, then going to university is a must. Adapting to life at university can be one of the most rewarding challenges you will ever face. Whatever subject you decide to study, going to university will equip you with skills that you can apply to your academic work, your career and in your personal life. The chance to nurture an academic passion over several years guided by an expert in that field, while simultaneously enjoying independence, extra-curricular activities and new friends is not to be easily overlooked.

If you're still not sure if university is right for you, talk to your teachers, speak with your family and friends, ask some students a few years above you to tell you their experiences and consider what it is you want to do for a career. Remember, this is a decision based on your aspirations and career dreams – put yourself and your feelings first. Think about the school subjects you enjoy and which classes you look forward to. In the end, however, the decision will be down to you. If you decide it's what you want, you'll need to fully understand the application process, select your course and pick your universities.

The benefits of Higher Education are endless – what you will learn both inside and outside of the lecture room will stay with you well beyond graduation day.

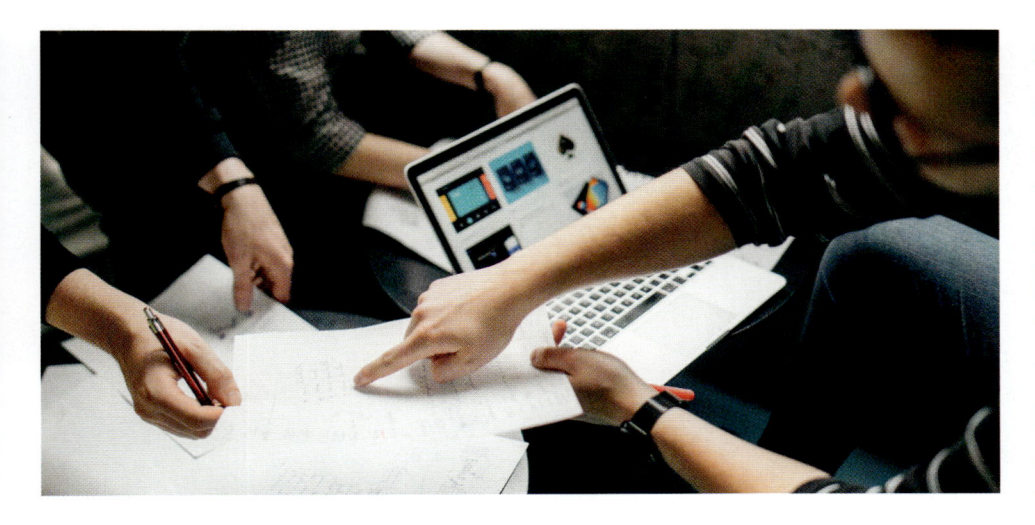

Immerse yourself in your chosen subject

Ever since you began your education, you probably had very little choice in the subjects you studied and the topics you covered, but university offers you the chance to explore a subject you are really interested in. Whether you choose a subject which you enjoy, a subject which you're good at - or both - university offers you the chance to study a subject of your choice for three years or more with guidance and tuition from experts in their fields, and in a place with excellent resources.

Enhance your career prospects

Getting a degree from a top university will enhance your career prospects in a number of ways. Employers like the commitment shown through studying one subject for three years. It also shows that you are able to work independently and are able to flourish in new, challenging environments (much like when you start a new job). Not only do you look highly attractive to employers because of your degree and the skills you develop along the way, but you will also increase your earning potential.

Expand your social life

Universities offer a whole host of new experiences which is often reflected in the lively nightlife of most university towns. That said, it's not all cheap beer and nights out; universities are a great place to meet like-minded people from all walks of life. It will offer you the chance to immerse yourself in a new culture and environment, and make friends with people who you may stay in touch with long after graduation.

Extra-curricular activities

Don't forget university is not just about studying! It is unlikely that you will ever have the opportunity to take part in such a wide range of activities as you will come across at university. You can join all sorts of clubs, societies and teams, from the usual things like football, debating and theatre to the fun things like belly-dancing, tea-drinking and Hollyoaks fan clubs. And the best thing of all is that if there isn't a society for what you love, then it's easy to start one yourself! Whatever your interests, you can pursue them in a social capacity and the increase in confidence and awareness you develop by spending time with different people through social and extra-curricular activities will often contribute to your education as much as your degree.

Gain independence

Whatever subject you decide to study, going to university will equip you with skills that you can apply to your academic work, your career and in your personal life. Independence is one of the key skills which you will develop whilst a student. Living and studying on your own will be totally different from your pre university life. To be able to study when you like, buy your own groceries, learn self-discipline and indulge yourself is something you may not have done before. You'll learn so much so fast – some of it the hard way but you'll have a great time laughing about it with your new friends. The university experience is to be grasped with both hands, to be appreciated as so much more than the venue of your studies.

"Studying maths at City University was definitely a worthwhile way to spend three years, it was a lot of hard work, trust me, but whilst working hard, I have been able to bank three years worth of valuable skills and knowledge which has been vital in securing a job."

"I picked a course which really reflected what I enjoyed & loved. Having the passion definitely made the late nights spent working on coursework and revising for exams that little bit easier."

"I was really unsure of what I wanted to study at university, so I decided to take a gap year, which was one of the best decisions I made! It helped me to gain some perspective on university and gave me some direction on what I wanted to study."

How to choose a course and uni

Choose a subject you enjoy

Generally speaking, you shouldn't pick a course you're good at over one you really love, because innate ability just isn't a match for passion in the long run. Ideally you will excel at the course you enjoy, but if you happen to have a gift for a subject but find it boring and uninspiring, then reconsider because you will have to motivate yourself to study in your own time at university and if that fundamental interest isn't there, you just won't do it!

What if I have never studied the subject before?

The great advantage of choosing a course based on something you studied at school is that you have an idea of what it involves, and you have a strong foundation of knowledge and skills to build on. That said, be aware that there's a lot of difference between the way a subject is taught in school and at university, or even the topics covered.

If you're interested in a subject that you either haven't studied at school, or wasn't available, then the onus is on you to discover everything you need to know to make sure it's right for you. There are over 37,000 courses on offer via UCAS, the highest in Europe, so there are plenty to choose from! Do some reading around your subject, the recommended reading lists on the university websites are a good place to start. As always, read the prospectus very carefully for information on how the course is taught and assessed.

Many universities offer a service where you can email students currently taking the course to ask them questions about their experiences. If you do decide to take a course you haven't studied before, don't worry if other students applying for the course have already taken the subject at school; the admissions tutor and syllabus will take account of these discrepancies, and you won't be behind for long.

UCAS tariff points

Once you've chosen your course you need to see if the grades you're expecting match up to the grade requirements. Every course on offer at any university will have an entry requirement which is set by the university. These can be found on both the university and UCAS websites. Different universities will set different entry requirements for the same subject. Think carefully about the requirements and be realistic when choosing your universities. If you are predicted 340 UCAS tariff points, and a university is asking for a minimum of 360, there is a chance your application will be unsuccessful. Wise students spread their choices across universities with a range of requirements to cover all eventualities come results day.

Career prospects

Are you absolutely certain what you want from your future career? If you are, then great, but many students find that their aspirations change between their teens and twenties. Though no-one can be absolutely certain of how their ambitions may shift, you should try to get some practical experience in the field you want to work in to check if it's for you. This will also help beef up your UCAS form.

If you are as sure as you can be, then perhaps you should consider a vocational course. A vocational course is one which is specifically designed to qualify you for a definitive career - for example, medicine, dentistry or nursing. If you are considering this kind of course, you should be aware of the pros and cons before you sign on the dotted line (or, in the case of the UCAS form, the submit button).

If you do have a career in mind, you must also love the idea of studying the subject theoretically. It doesn't matter how committed you are to becoming a lawyer, you will find yourself falling behind your peers if you do not love the academic disciplines of law because the academic study of the subject is very different to its practical application. You should also check if it really is necessary to study that subject to pursue a career in that field – for example, lawyers are NOT required to study law, and you don't have to study finance or economics to work in the financial sector.

The law conversion course (GDL) and the medical fast track programme are two examples of post-graduate courses which allow you to catch up on all the stuff that everyone else did during their degree. Many employers value the breadth of knowledge which people who did different degrees at university can bring to their professions.

If, like most students, you are not sure yet, or have absolutely no idea then just choose a course that you find interesting and keep your options open.

Questions to ask yourself

Remember that no single person or organisation, not even UCAS, can be an expert on all courses or universities. It is up to you to do your own research for the most up-to-date facts.

You'll want to consider what is most important to you. A good reputation? New facilities? Near to home or as far away as possible? A tight-knit community, or large campus? In a city, or a leafy campus? Spacious accommodation, or shared rooms? What's the local nightlife like? Is it safe? Do you have to share bathrooms, or are they en suite? High employment statistics and a great careers service? Is the accommodation catered, or will you have to cook for yourself? How far away is your local supermarket or bank? How much will it cost you to travel between home and university? Does the library have good facilities like online journals and e-books? Are there a broad range of societies? Can you get involved in theatre? How about sport?

Prospectuses, university league tables, and UCAS are all useful resources in helping to answer these questions, but nothing beats an open day which allows you to get a feel for a place.

Although practical considerations can make a big difference to your university years, you're going away to study, and ultimately the content of the course should be your guiding principle, no matter how much fun Freshers' Week sounds, or how many nightclubs the town has! Create your own league table based on the factors that are most important to you.

Don't be influenced by where friends are headed – people can have very different priorities when choosing universities and one of the most wonderful things about university life are the new friends that you will make.

ARE YOU QUALIFIED?

Don't waste one of your five precious choices on a course you're not qualified to do! In addition to grade requirements some courses require specific A-Levels, extra qualifications or experience – make sure you've checked. If you're not sure of something, call the university admissions office to check.

HAVE YOU LOOKED INTO IT FULLY?

Course choice is consistently the top reason why students drop out of uni in the first year so make sure that you have researched extensively and are confident you know what you are in for. Every course will approach the subject from a different angle. For instance, if you take French at Oxford, you will find yourself reading a great deal of French literature. Take the French course at Newcastle and there'll be a lot less literature, but a lot more language and sociology.

HAVE YOU SELECTED SIMILAR COURSES?

Make sure the five courses you select are similar to each other - you only get to submit one personal statement, so you'll have a hard job convincing an admissions tutor you're interested in economics but also zoology. The only exception here is for medical applications, you can have a course such as biomedical sciences as back-up. Read more on healthcare in the career profiles section.

WHAT ARE THE DIFFERENT ROUTES AVAILABLE?

It can be easy to get swept up in the standard UCAS process that it seems everyone else is doing, but there are alternative options out there that could be right for you such as part-time study, apprenticeships, distance learning, working while gaining a degree. For more on degree apprenticeships or school leaver programmes, see the alternatives to uni section.

HAVE YOU BEEN TO THE CAMPUS?

Visit as many open days as you can – you will never get 'the feel' of a place just through reading a glossy prospectus. Speak to lots of current students whilst you're there – they will be able to give you that all-important insider knowledge. You should also look into summer schools and insight days – many universities offer students the chance to stay on-campus, attending talks by lecturers and exploring the course.

University league tables
(and how to use them)

University league tables can be a useful tool to use when choosing your future place of study. You can find plenty of them online, but with different tables ranking universities in different orders, it's important to find out what factors are involved, and consider how much attention you should be paying to them.

Useful facts to know

DEGREES OF SEPARATION

According to the Higher Education Liaison Officers Association, you shouldn't read too much into universities that are five or ten places apart on the league table. A university in 20th place is usually separated from one in 30th place by only a few percentage points.

CHANGING PLACES

Universities that are right at the top of the league tables are obviously doing well according to all of the relevant criteria. However, the top of the league tables is consistently dominated by Oxford and Cambridge, LSE and Imperial. It might be worth looking more carefully at those universities which have dropped or risen dramatically compared with their position in the last few years and finding out why.

SUBJECT RANKING

It is also useful to look at how the subject ranks, not just the institution as a whole. Some universities have particularly strong faculties that are internationally famous, even if the institution itself may be lower on the league tables. Look out for these types of courses and make sure you do your research, particularly in specialist areas. The results can be very surprising, for example Glasgow is currently number 27 on the Complete University Guide's table, however their law faculty is rated number 5 in the country.

A GOOD FIT FOR YOU

Choosing the right course for you is ultimately the most important thing. Looking at league tables does not replace the need for you to thoroughly research available modules, course structure and assessment methods. Other factors like the distance from your home to university, entry requirements and long-term career options are also very important. Attending university open days can be a really good way of finding out whether a university suits you.

FUTURE EMPLOYERS

Employers will also use university league tables when assessing which candidates to select from. Try to apply to at least one or two universities that consistently appear in the top 50 – they are likely to be the ones held in higher regard by future employers.

Be aware

STUDENT SATISFACTION

The student satisfaction score can show you what current students think about their university experience. Bear in mind that this percentage might not just be based on the university's academics but on their experience as a whole, and that scores don't vary that much between different universities.

STUDENT TO STAFF RATIO

This gives you an idea of how much money a university invests in its staffing. This does not necessarily tell you how many hours of teaching you personally will get, or who will be teaching you.

GRADUATE PROSPECTS

These scores can tell you what graduates go on to do after university. Statistics are collected six months after graduation, so can sometimes give you a skewed idea of what the graduate prospects actually are.

ENTRY GRADES

Normally the league table will show what the average UCAS tariff was for each student starting at the specific institution. Most students' UCAS tariff is usually higher than the course requirements, and so it can make it look like some universities are out of reach. Make sure you always look at the university's individual course requirements, rather than relying on the tariff scores produced by the league tables.

USEFUL RESOURCES	
	thecompleteuniversityguide.co.uk
	timeshighereducation.co.uk
	theguardian.com/education

MANCHESTER 1824
The University of Manchester

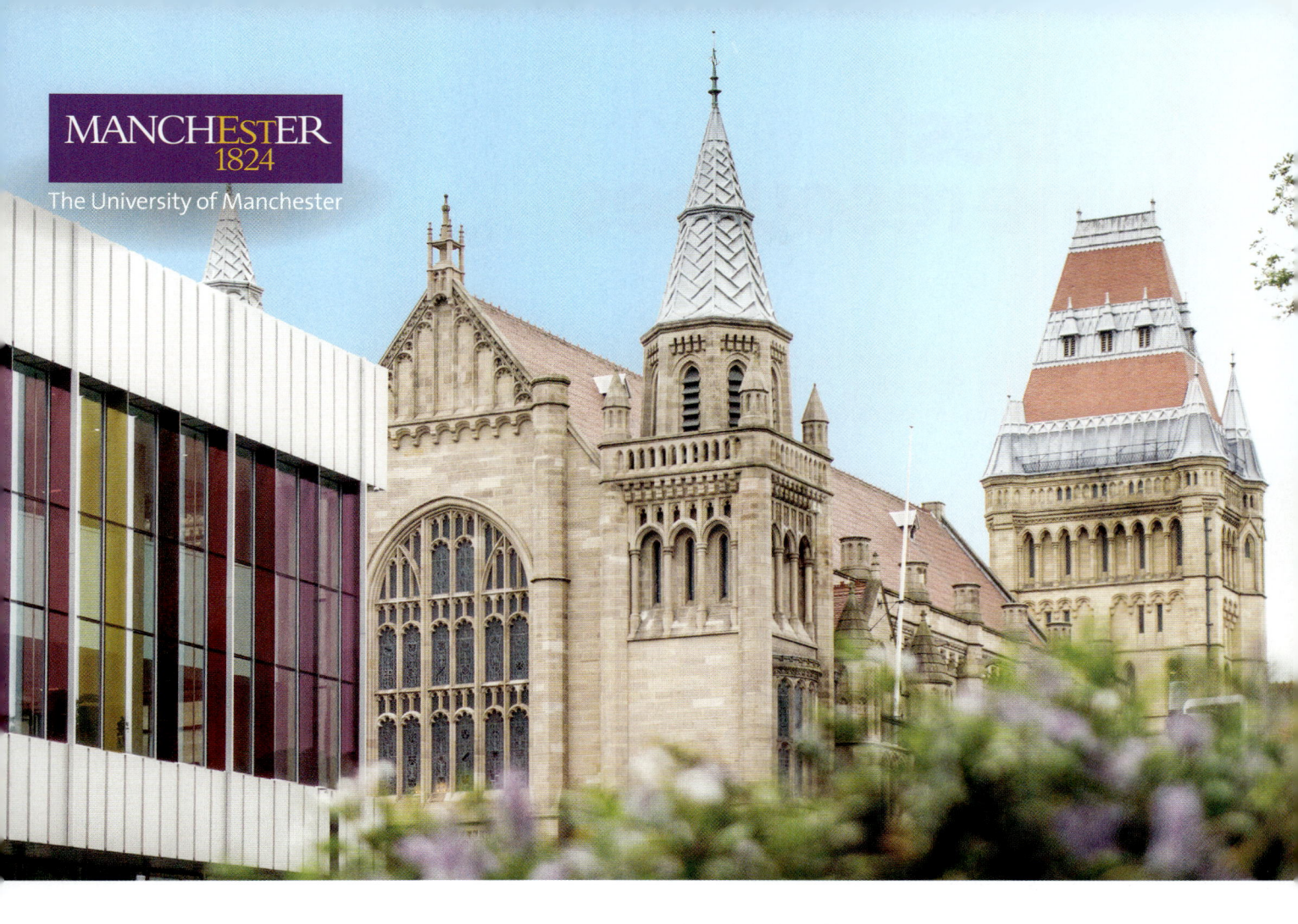

MANCHESTER

With over 400 courses, The University of Manchester offers something for everyone. Find out which course is for you by visiting the course search website:

🖥 www.manchester.ac.uk/undergraduate/courses

Undergraduate Open Days

Come and get a feel for life at the UK's largest single-site university at one of our Open Days.

- Friday, 22 June 2018
- Saturday, 23 June 2018
- Saturday, 29 September 2018
- Saturday, 13 October 2018

Financial support

If you've got the ability, finance shouldn't be a barrier to success. Each year a third of all new home undergraduate students benefit from our Manchester Bursary.

🖥 www.manchester.ac.uk/studentfinance

University of Manchester Aspiring Students Society (UMASS)

UMASS is for Year 12, Year 13 and Access to HE students who are considering going to university. UMASS gives you an insight into university life and advice on the application process.

🖥 www.umass.manchester.ac.uk

Access Manchester

We offer a range of access schemes for Year 12 and 13 students which help to increase your preparedness for university.

🖥 www.access.manchester.ac.uk

The best online resources

Choosing your university can be a daunting prospect but the wonderful World Wide Web is a great place to start. Spending a little time doing online research can enable you to eliminate certain courses and universities and start to hone in on the ones that are going to be the right fit for you.

USE ONLINE TOOLS

An obvious place to start is the UCAS website which will give you information about which university runs which courses. But there are also a host of other sites that are specifically geared to help you dig a little deeper. WhatUni? lets you filter your results to look for a specific module you're interested in or prioritise universities that are a certain distance from your home postcode. Similarly, 'Which? University' enables you to filter by your predicted grades and create your own 'shortlist' as you look through different courses. You can even sign up to 'Which? University' alerts for tips and advice about decision making and reminders of upcoming deadlines.

CHECK OUT ONLINE RANKINGS

The internet is a great place to look at all of the major university league tables and compare their rankings. Check out websites such as: 'The Complete University Guide'.

FIND OUT WHAT CURRENT STUDENTS THINK

Community sites like The Student Room allow you to get involved in discussions with current students, ask any questions you may have, and read about other peoples' personal experiences of applying to university.

It's also worth checking out the student satisfaction rankings that help make up university league tables and reading some student reviews of universities (WhatUni? has loads on their website).

FIND OUT MORE ABOUT LOCATION

It's important not to forget to give due consideration to location when choosing your uni. Once you've narrowed your choices down a little, a quick Google Maps search will be able to give you an indication of how long it will take you to get back home and doing some basic online research should enable you to start to build a picture of the area – how safe it is, how urban or rural, how new or historic, how far the uni facilities are from the nearest town or city.

OPEN DAYS (BOTH VIRTUAL + REALITY)

We understand that it might not be logistically possible to get along to the open day of every single one of the universities that you're interested in – this is where virtual tours can help. UCAS now has a nifty bit of their website with links to virtual open days at most of the big universities. Watching these can give you a 'feel' for the university and help you to narrow down which ones you might want to actually visit in person.

Once you've decided which universities you want to pay a visit to it is a good idea to do some planning. Universities will have details of upcoming open days on their websites and you will normally be able to book onto these online. Make sure to check out the rest of the website so that you head to the open day armed with any questions you may wish to ask.

TWITTER

Almost all universities now have a range of affiliated Twitter accounts, for their departments, their careers service, their student union, etc. which you can follow to keep up to date with news and events. Doing so can provide a useful insight into the day-to-day activities of a university and help you work out which universities are doing stuff that's of most interest to you. You can also follow lecturers from the university to stay informed with progress in their fields – this can be particularly useful for keeping in touch with your subject of choice and making sure you're ready for any potential academic interviews.

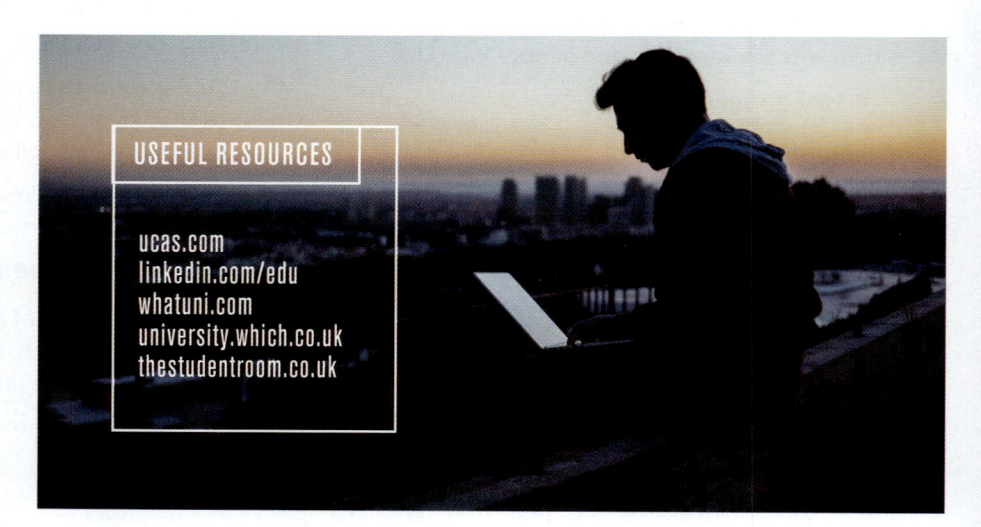

USEFUL RESOURCES

ucas.com
linkedin.com/edu
whatuni.com
university.which.co.uk
thestudentroom.co.uk

Imperial College London

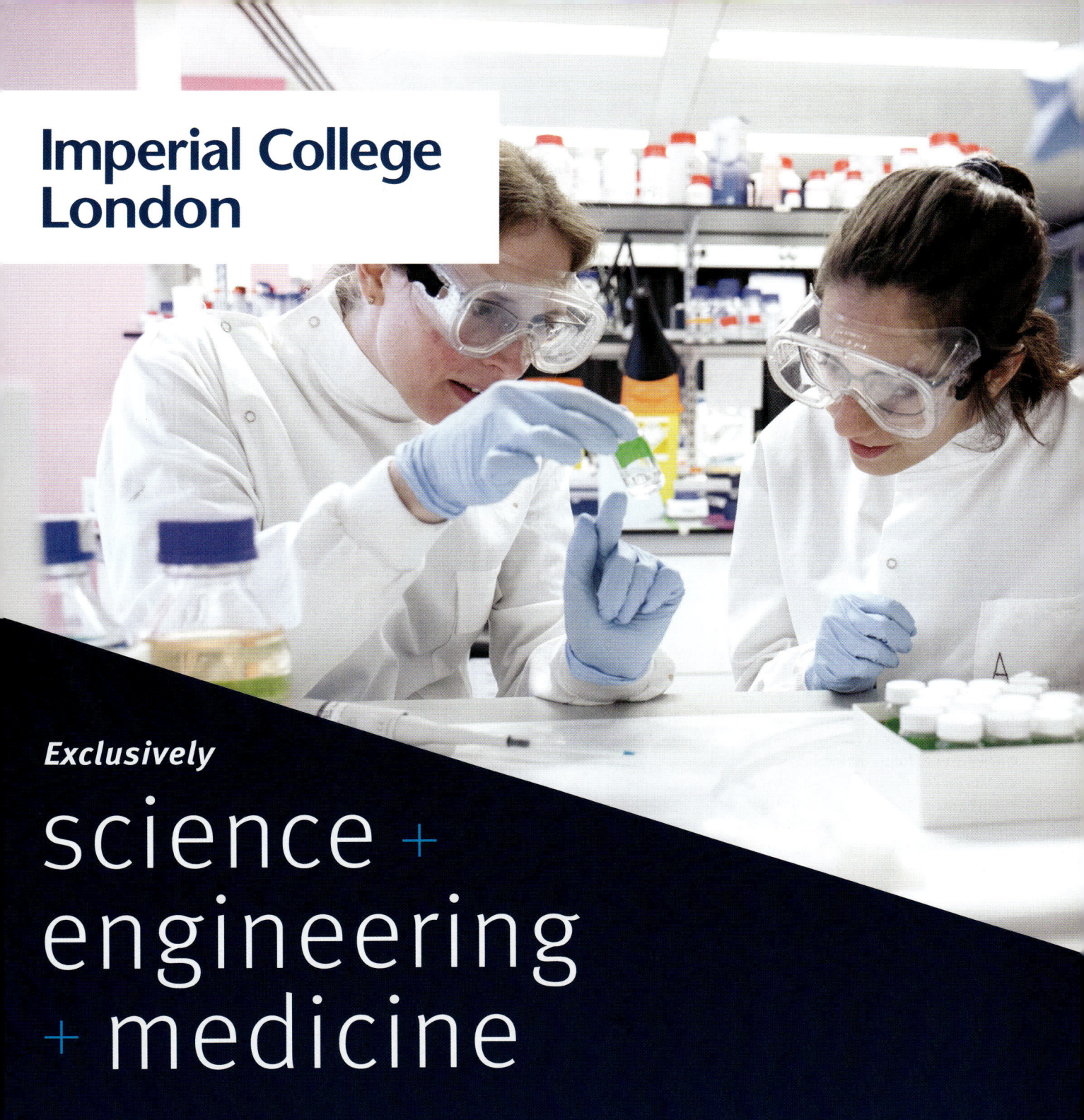

Exclusively

science + engineering + medicine

Top 10 best university in the world

The Times Higher Education World University Rankings 2018

No.1 in the UK for graduate salaries

The Times and Sunday Times Good University Guide 2018

WWW.IMPERIAL.AC.UK/STUDY/UG

University open days

Choosing which university to go to out of so many options can be an extremely daunting prospect but open days can really help. They are a brilliant way to find out more about a university, see the place for yourself and make a decision.

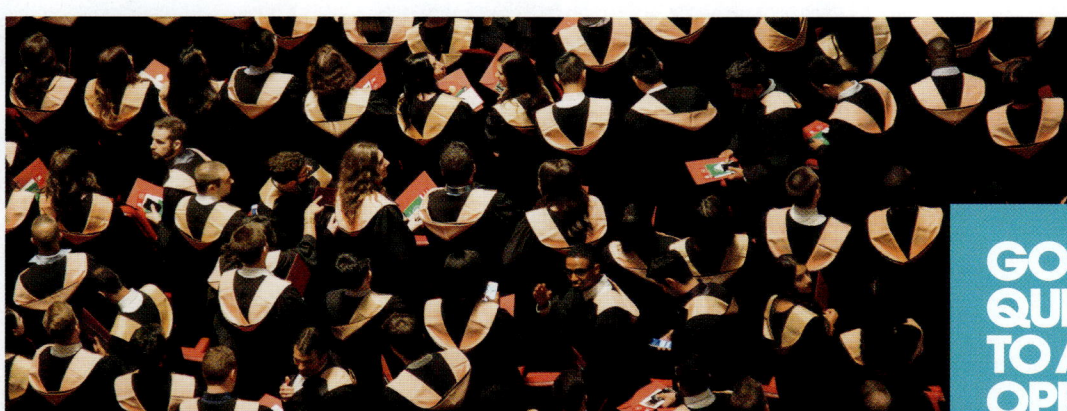

In order to get the most out of your visit and ensure you get the information you need to make the right decision, you will need to do some preparation beforehand. Make sure you've at least researched the university and found out if they offer the course you're after and grade requirements you can meet – don't waste time visiting and falling in love with a university that you're not going to be able to get into. Better still, check out the course structure and make sure you find it appealing.

PLAN AHEAD

Most universities will include a timetable of what lectures, talks and events will be going on during the day on their website. Make sure you take a look at this and plan your day to maximise what you can find out about and ensure you don't miss any of the key things you've travelled there for.

GO ARMED WITH LOTS OF QUESTIONS

And make sure you ask them! There's no point driving miles and miles to visit a university just to sit quietly through a sample lecture, grab a prospectus and head home. Make sure to talk to the staff who will be leading your course, interrogate some current students about how they're finding the experience and visit the people working at the careers service, the sports facilities and the student support services to find out more about what's on offer from each. Open days are a great opportunity to ask any of those burning questions that haven't been answered in the prospectus. Use the opportunity to check out the range of accommodation options. Universities use open days to try and sell themselves and as such it's likely you'll be shown the nicest lecture halls and taken to see the best accommodation on campus. Try, where possible, to get a good look at the whole of the campus and all of the different accommodation types on offer.

VENTURE INTO THE NEAREST TOWN OR CITY

You'll be spending a lot of time there if you go to that university so it's important that you like it and feel comfortable in it.

USEFUL RESOURCES

www.opendays.com
www.ucas.com
www.whatuni.com

GOOD QUESTIONS TO ASK AT AN OPEN DAY:

What will you be doing as part of your course on a weekly basis?

How many hours of contact will you have?

What's the balance between practice and theory?

Are there opportunities to study abroad as part of the course you're interested in?

Could you study a joint or combined course?

Are all the buildings on campus or are they spread over a town?

Can you choose different modules during your course?

What clubs and societies does the university have?

What kind of social life is there?

Is there night life on campus?

LONDON'S GLOBAL UNIVERSITY

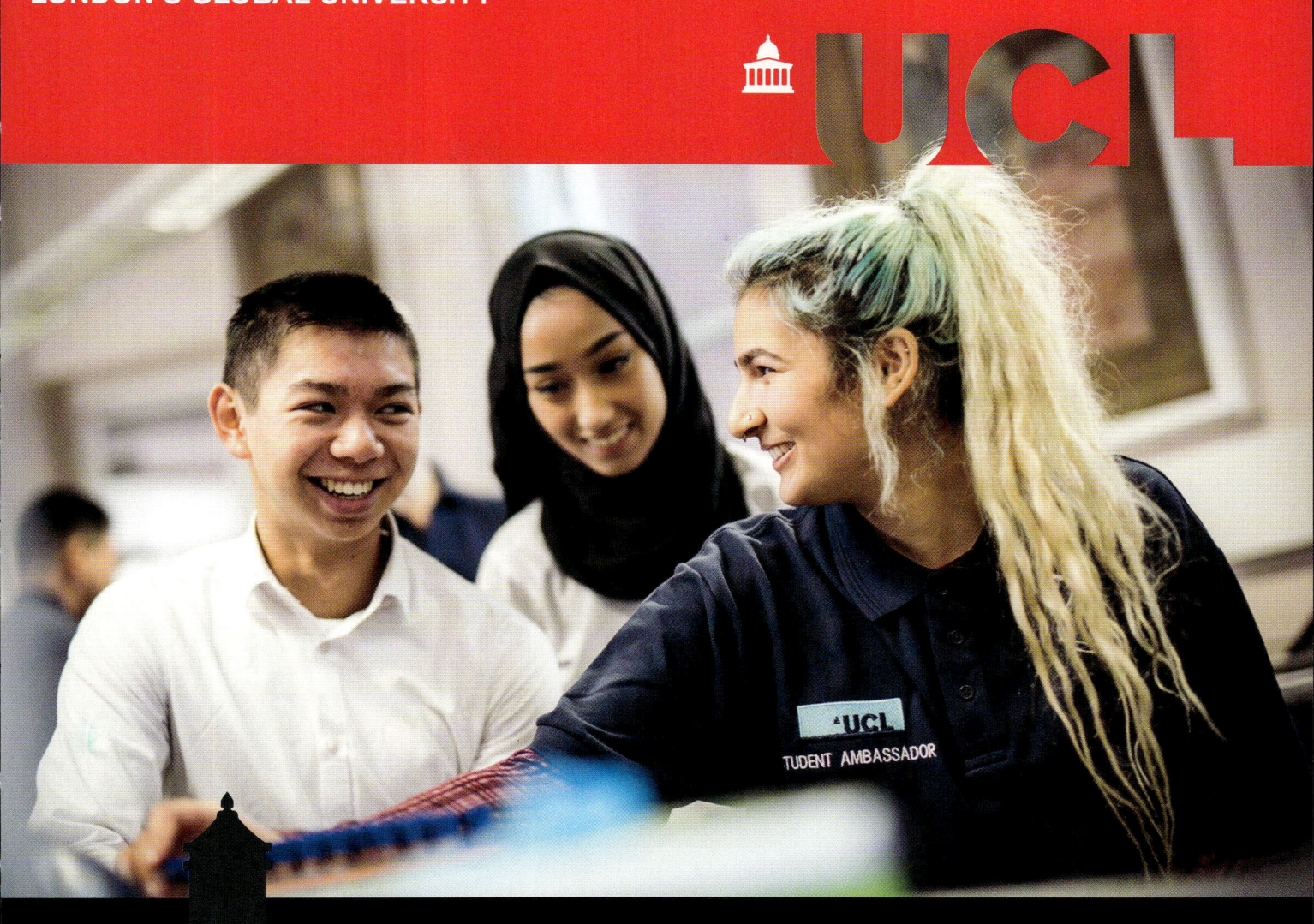

UCL

Discover your future at UCL

Ranked among the world's best universities (2016/17 QS World University), UCL's degree programmes will equip you to think critically and creatively in preparation for your career.

We offer a huge range of subjects spanning the arts, humanities, sciences, engineering, built environment and more.

Find out more about your options and UCL through our taster activities.

For further information and advice for students, parents and teachers follow us on social media:

- Discover UCL
- discoverucl
- DiscoverUCL
- @DiscoverUCL

www.ucl.ac.uk/wp

#

Applying to Oxford or Cambridge

The universities of Oxford and Cambridge, sometimes collectively referred to as Oxbridge, are internationally famous for their research, their excellent teaching and the quality of their graduates.

Are you consistently at the top of your class?

Are you on course for A or A* grades at A-Level?

Did you get excellent GCSE grades?

Do you enjoy reading about your chosen subject in your own time?

Does the stuff you learn at school or college inspire you to do your own research?

Do you find that your school work throws up questions that you would like to devote more time trying to answer?

Do you enjoy discussing your views with classmates, parents and teachers?

As well as having extraordinary resources, both materially and in the expertise of their staff, they practice something called the tutorial (at Oxford) or supervision (at Cambridge) system. This means that in addition to the normal course of lectures, students will spend two hours per week individually or in very small groups, discussing their work with a world-class academic in their field. This not only allows students to develop their written work, but also encourages the development of confidence and verbal fluency. Furthermore, both universities are made up of a number of smaller colleges, which means that settling in is much easier than other universities. For that reason each college will be able to provide a very high level of academic and pastoral care to each student. It may also be of great interest to learn that the terms are much shorter than other universities (8 weeks compared to 10-12 weeks) but are considerably more intense!

Oxbridge graduates enjoy unparalleled career prospects, and having one of these universities on your CV will impress employers, and stand you in good stead for the rest of your career. Many of the top employers visit Oxbridge finalists to try and recruit them early on, as they recognise the value of the skills students have developed during their studies.

The application process is more rigorous than many other universities, but don't let this put you off – they are looking for bright, ambitious students with lots of potential, whatever their social or economic background. Don't be distracted by the myths surrounding Oxbridge either. Oxford and Cambridge are teaching institutions just like anywhere else and all they are looking for is the sharpest young minds available to study their subjects.

WHO ARE THEY LOOKING FOR?

Nearly everybody goes to Oxbridge worrying that they won't be as clever as all their new classmates, and each new student discovers that the image of a university filled with geniuses is entirely a media illusion. Equally, Oxford and Cambridge are not full of posh people punting down rivers. The majority of students (around 60%) come from state schools and both universities are taking active measures to encourage applications from non-traditional backgrounds. Look into the Oxford and Cambridge Access Schemes on their websites.

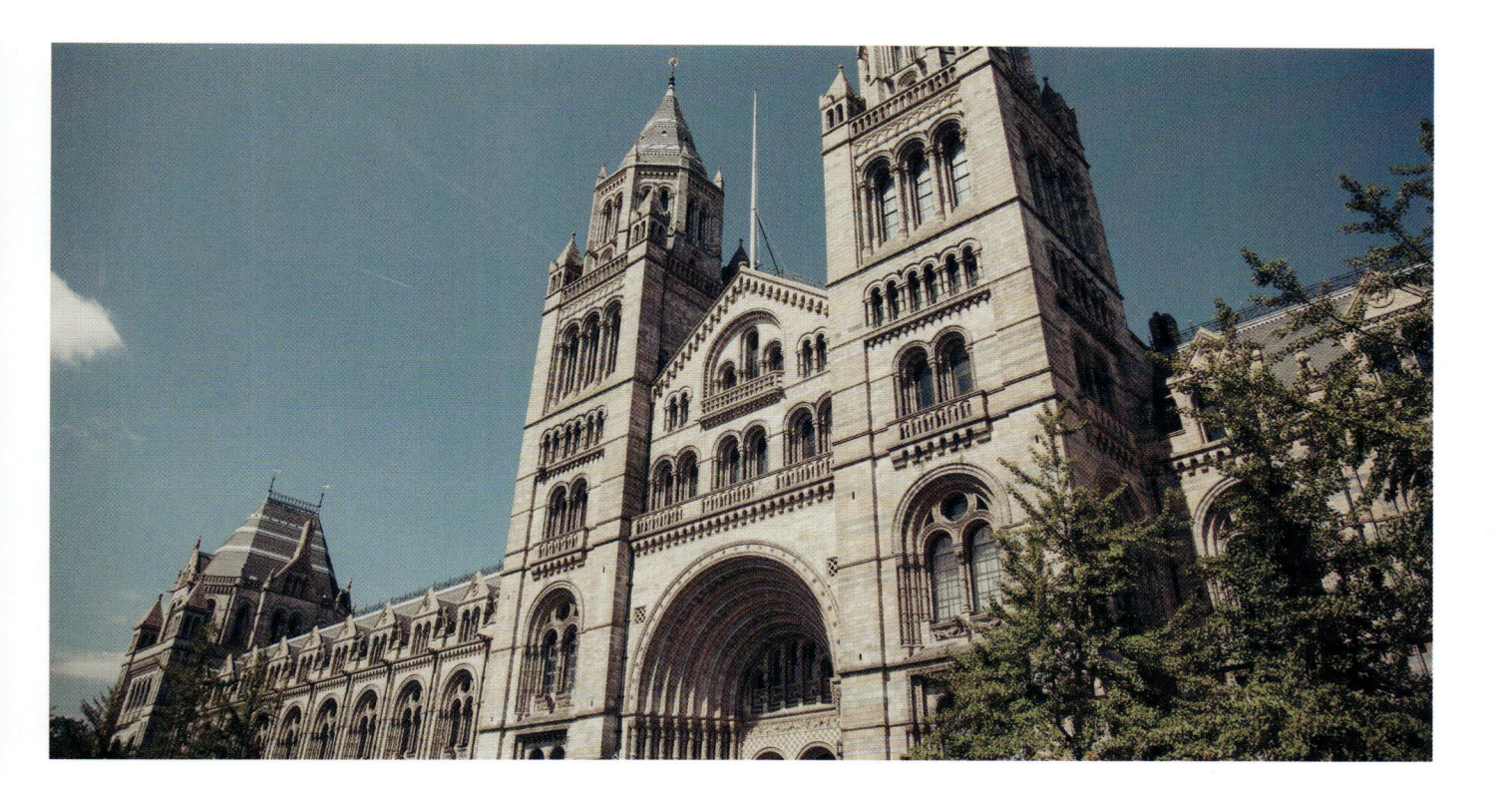

SHOULD I APPLY TO OXFORD OR CAMBRIDGE?

You cannot apply to both, so you need to pick one. In reality, there is very little difference between the two institutions and both have the same academic reputation. You can also apply to up to four other universities.

THE APPLICATION PROCESS

The deadline for applications to both Oxford and Cambridge is October 15th, so ideally you should be working on your personal statement throughout the summer holiday after Year 12, so that you are ready to send off your application come October.

HOW DO I CHOOSE A COLLEGE?

Both universities are made up of around 30-40 colleges, and you can apply directly to the college of your choice.

Each college holds its own open day, often in conjunction with the main university open day. It might be a good idea to attend a few of these to get more of a feel of what life at the college could be like. Alternatively, the colleges are usually open to the public every day except in the examination period, so if you are unable to attend the prescribed open day it is possible to visit on a day that suits you.

If you are finding it difficult to choose a college, you can do what is called an open application. The university will then allocate you a college at random. Your application will not be negatively affected by choosing this route.

FACTORS TO CONSIDER WHEN CHOOSING A COLLEGE

SUBJECT
Whether your chosen degree course is offered at the college.

SIZE
Colleges usually range between about 60 and 200 students per year group.

LOCATION
The cities of Oxford and Cambridge are both relatively small, especially since most colleges are located in the city centre. Living five minutes away from your lectures, the university sports pitches, the town centre or Sainsbury's is convenient. A lot of students choose to cycle whilst at university, so journeys are usually very short.

APPEARANCE
Would you prefer to attend an old college or a more modern one?

ACCOMMODATION
Is it offered for all three years?

GENDER
If you are female, there are some all-girls colleges that you might consider applying to.

FACILITIES
Some colleges will have their own sports pitches, theatres, cinemas, music practice rooms and chapels, for example.

STRENGTHS
Is the college renowned for music, sport, drama etc.?

SCHOLARSHIPS & BURSARIES
Are you considering applying for a choral, sport or instrumental scholarship? Check to see whether the college of your choice offers these awards. Many colleges also offer bursaries and hardship funds.

ACADEMIC STAFF
Does the Director of Studies or other Fellows at the college match your own academic interests?

What happens after I submit my application?

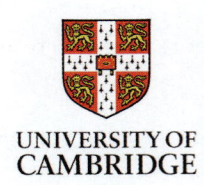

If you applied to Cambridge…

You will be asked to fill in an online form (the Supplementary Application Questionnaire, SAQ). You will have to supply your year 12 (or equivalent) exam results module results and answer a few other questions about your experience so far and possible career paths. You are not expected to know what you want to do after graduation at this point.

If your application is successful, you will be invited for interview, which normally takes place at the beginning of December. The interview process is different for each subject, so you must check the college website for guidelines on what to expect. Normally you will have about three interviews lasting roughly twenty minutes each. There is no typical Cambridge interview, but you will definitely be asked further questions on what you wrote in your personal statement, and what you have studied so far in your A-Level course. You should be well prepared for obvious questions such as 'why Cambridge?' and 'why your chosen subject?'. You might also be given a short test beforehand or during the interview. It is easy to be put off by horror stories surrounding the Oxbridge interview process. The interviews are difficult, but they are also your chance to speak to a leading expert in your subject. The interviewers will push you as hard as they can, and if you cannot answer a question that does not necessarily mean that you have failed the interview stage. They are much more interested in your potential than your current knowledge.

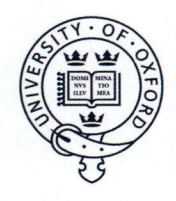

If you applied to Oxford…

The Oxford application process is very similar. The only difference is that for Oxford, there is no extra application form to fill in, so the university does not see your year 12 (or equivalent) exam results. Instead, most subjects require their applicants to sit a short test before they choose which candidates will progress to the interview stage. These tests are normally taken at your school. Again, it is important to check the department and college websites for details specific to your subject. The same interview advice applies for applications to Oxford. It is the norm for students applying to Oxford to spend a few days and stay overnight in the college. Accommodation and food are provided free of charge by the college, and social events are organised for the evenings.

You will be notified of either university's decision in December or January, the exact timings vary depending on which faculty you applied to.

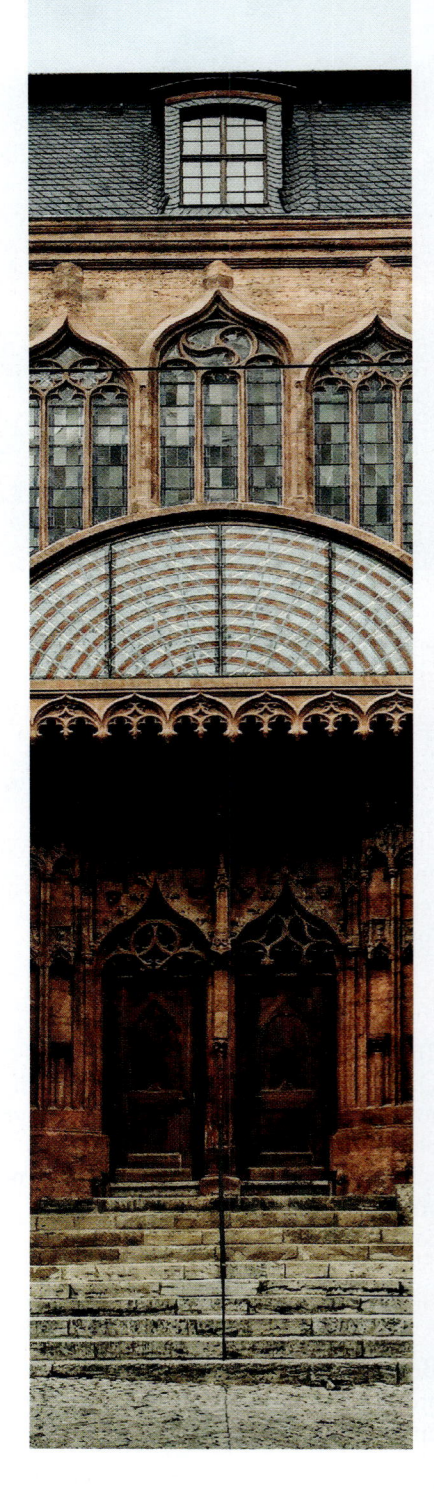

USEFUL RESOURCES

ox.ac.uk
cam.ac.uk
thestudentroom.co.uk

My Experience Applying to Oxford

By Madeleine Hayes
(4th from left)

"It's easy to think that just because you come from a more disadvantaged background than most that you should set your aspirations low or at most just do what is expected of you. I did exactly the opposite. Applying to Oxford from a state school in the Midlands I inevitably had concerns. Firstly, though my Sixth Form was of a good standard, only one or two people got in to Oxbridge each year. Secondly, neither of my parents went to Oxford or had studied or practised Law. While these concerns could have made me not bother with the application process all together, I decided to take every opportunity given to me to find out more about whether Oxford Law was right for me.

In the March of Year 12 I attended a Law Masterclass at Cambridge University, advertised through my school. The day consisted of four or five lectures on various legal topics. It was a fantastic insight into what challenges would be debated through the study of Law at degree. Whilst I left confident that studying Law was right for me, I was slightly put off from applying to Cambridge. The vast majority of people sat with me were from the South and my bland Midlands accent stuck out like a sore thumb.

Another opportunity I heard about was the UNIQ Law Summer School. I applied by submitting a short personal statement and my GCSE grades. The week long scheme is an access initiative run by Oxford University Law Faculty and aims to increase applications to Oxford from students with low socio-economic status or from areas with low progression to higher education. During UNIQ, I attended masterclasses, lectures and workshops on many areas of Law giving a good insight into what you should expect from a Law degree, particularly having never studied Law myself. The best part of UNIQ for me was meeting like-minded individuals, exploring the beautiful city of Oxford, getting advice from alumni at formal dinners and having fun at a bop (an Oxford party!). It proved to me that the stereotypes about Oxford aren't true and I had a shot at getting a place.

The next step for me was going to the Oxford Open Day. I'd already made up my mind that I wanted to apply but I needed to pick a college (you apply to one college rather than the university as a whole) and my mum also needed convincing that I would fit in. I completed an online questionnaire that ranks which colleges would be best for you based on questions like 'how important is being close to the centre for you?' and began looking around each. After looking at seven, I reached Jesus College and it just felt right. The friendly students showing me round in their green jumpers. They didn't look down at me or question if I was an 'Oxford fit'… because in all honesty there is no Oxford type. Everyone at Jesus College was different and I liked that.

Once I applied to Jesus College for Law it was an anxious wait to find out if I'd been invited to interview… but luckily I had! The letter from the College Principal arrived in the post, inviting me to stay at Jesus College for two or three days and have at least two interviews.

During the interviews, any statement I made was challenged but I never felt intimidated or pressured. The tutors wanted to know how I think and whether I would be right for the tutorial system. For me, I left each interview feeling like I'd done my best - that's all you can give! It was a long wait until January when another letter arrived in the post with the decision on whether I was to be offered a conditional place…. I WAS! I was beyond proud of myself that I beat all the odds and was soon to embark on something that would genuinely change my life (once I got the 3 As needed at A-Level!). The College invited offer holders to a special day in February where we would meet each other and talk to current students ahead of sitting our A-Level exams. As I looked around the room it was clear that everyone truly was unique. We all came from different backgrounds, had different opportunities and yet were to be studying at what (that year) became the number 1 university in the world!

Now in my second year of studying Law at Oxford I am amazed at how much I have achieved. From being a fresh-faced girl from the East Midlands, who was the only person to get a place at Oxford out of 300 students in my year, I am the Vice-President Elect of Oxford Law Society, the Kit and Social Secretary (as well as a player) for Oxford University Korfball Club and Captain of three College sports… all while achieving a 2.1 in my first year exams!

As an advocate for improving access and widening participation in the legal sector, I am also a Linklaters Oxford Law Access Ambassador and this summer was a Team Leader on the Pathways to Law National Conference. I am keen to encourage everyone to take at shot at applying to Oxford.

I am now embarking on a new challenge… breaking the glass ceiling and fighting the lack of diversity in Commercial Law!"

Applying through UCAS

If you decide that university is right for you, and you have chosen your course and the universities you'd like to study at, you will have to fill in an application. All applications are handled through a centralised agency, the University and Colleges Admissions Service (UCAS), which has over 380 member institutions. Almost everyone will apply through UCAS and not directly to the university concerned.

You can apply individually or through your school (most students apply via their school to get that additional support). If you're applying as an individual, you will need to answer a few simple questions to confirm your eligibility before you can start your application. If applying through your school or college, they will issue you with a unique 'buzzword' which enables UCAS to link you to your school.

You can fill the form in stages and make changes as you go along, just make sure you don't pay the fee until you are completely ready:

Sections of the UCAS form

PERSONAL DETAILS
This section will ask for your name (as it appears on your passport), address, date of birth, nationality, residential status (e.g. EU citizen), passport details and any special needs. You will be asked to create your own password and answer four security questions. Make a note of your username, password and your personal ID, and keep it in a safe place.

NOMINATED ACCESS
if you want to, you can give the details of a nominated person who can look at your application and also make decisions on your behalf, such as a parent or guardian.

ADDITIONAL INFORMATION
Here, you will be asked to state your ethnic origin and the occupation of your parents. This information is used by UCAS and other organisations for research on the demographic make-up of university applicants and not for selection purposes. You will also have the opportunity to include any activities you have participated in to prepare for Higher Education. Summer schools would be ideal for this, as would campus visits, summer academies, taster courses or widening participation activities. This does not include open days and if you haven't done anything, then leave it blank.

STUDENT SUPPORT
Students in the UK will have to fill in this section. This isn't your actual student finance application, but filling in this part of the form will speed up the application process for when you apply for student finance.

COURSE CHOICES
The majority of students can make applications through UCAS to up to five courses. You can select just one course, but this is unusual and risky. There are some exceptions. For example, applicants for Medicine, Dentistry, Veterinary Science or Veterinary Medicine can apply for no more than four of these courses and if you decide you want to go to Oxford or Cambridge, you have to choose between the two, though you can still put down other universities. Check UCAS if you are unsure.

This section of the form requires you to list each of the universities and courses applied for. The universities appear in alphabetical order, not by order of preference. When the individual universities look at your application, they will NOT be able to see which other universities you have applied to. Each institution and course has a code, which can be found on the UCAS website and you will have to state if you will be living at home or in student accommodation.

EDUCATION SECTION
Fill in your exam results so far and the exams you plan to take. You will have to enter all qualifications, even if you are retaking, awaiting your exam results or if you got unsuccessful grades.

EMPLOYMENT SECTION
You will be asked to give details of any employment to date. This includes weekend and holiday jobs.

PERSONAL STATEMENT
We'll look at this rather daunting aspect of the form in detail later in this section.

REFERENCE
After completing all of the above, you have to send the whole document online to your referee (a teacher) so he or she can confirm the accuracy of the details you've given. The referee is there to comment on your academic achievement and potential, suitability and motivation. They also help the admission tutors assess your personal

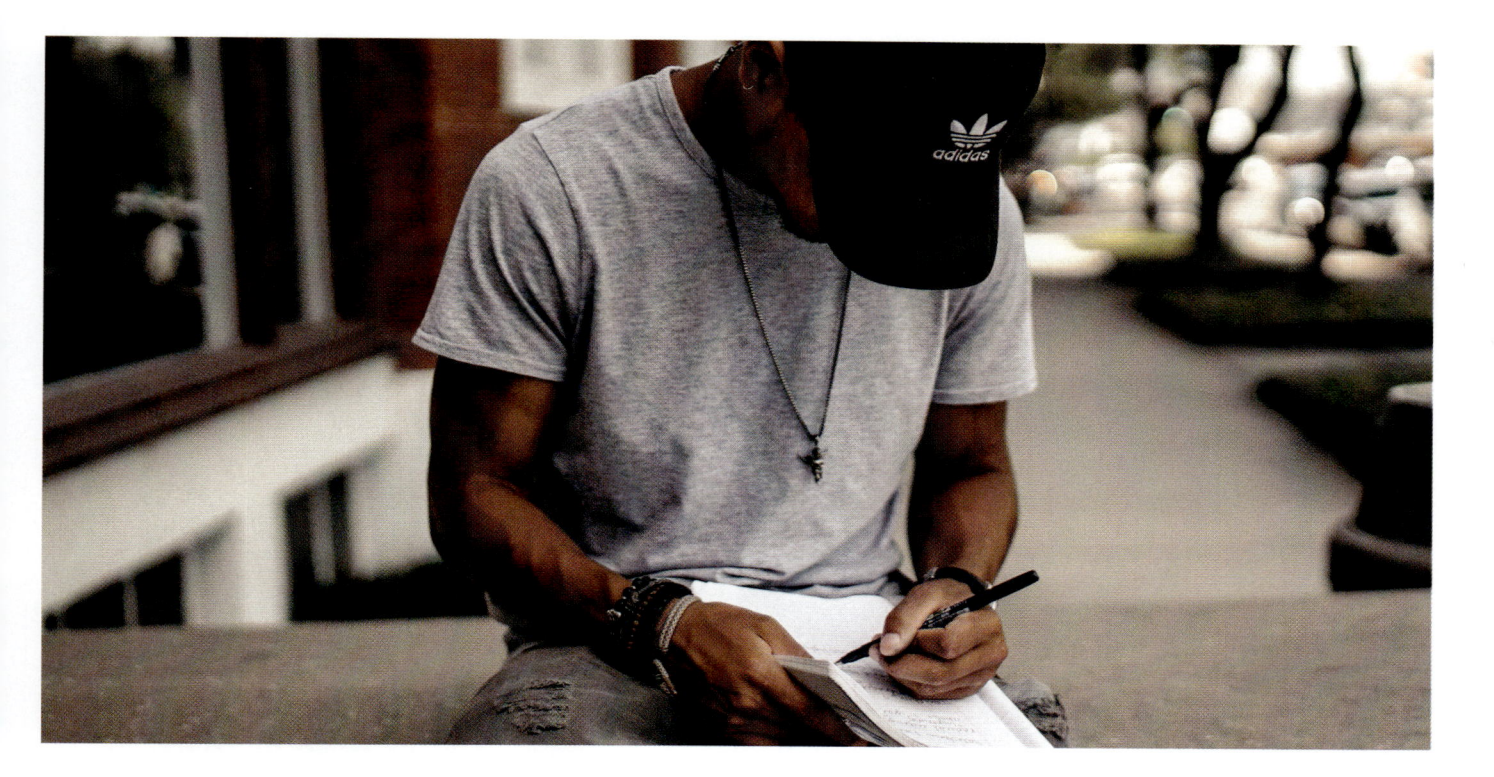

qualities, career aspirations and exam predictions. Make sure you ask your teacher about your reference as early as possible – they're likely to be writing a lot!

DEFERRED ENTRY
If you are deferring your entry to university, please note that the same deadlines apply for submitting your UCAS application. You will still need to make your choices, but remember to check with the university whether you are able to defer your entry. In fact, some universities may not offer the course the following year, so make sure you check. Note that maths applicants are not encouraged to take this option and in some cases refused… speak to your chosen institutions to find out the score.

PAYMENT
UCAS have a fee for processing each application and this amount is dependent on how many universities you are applying to. They charge £24 to apply to more than one university, and £13 to apply for one course at one university. Your school will send you more information about how to go about paying this fee so hold tight until then. If you feel that you are unable to pay this fee, speak with your teachers and they will be able to give you advice. It is worth noting that there is a 14-day cooling-off period within which you are entitled to a refund if you decide against applying to university.

Once you have filled everything in to your satisfaction, you will then pay for the application which will enable your teacher to add the reference. Once this has been completed, your school/college will then submit it electronically. UCAS will then process it for you and pass your application on to the universities you applied to.

Anomalies

ADDITIONAL QUALIFICATIONS
Sometimes you will need to provide further evidence of your suitability for the course, for example:

– Art & Design or Performing Arts applicants may need to attend an audition or submit a portfolio (there may be a fee for this).
– You may have to send in an essay or written piece of work.
– You might be called for interview. An increasing number of universities are calling students to interview in addition to the UCAS form. This shouldn't put you off but you need to be prepared, so do your research.
– Some will require an admissions test.

Places at top university courses have become increasingly competitive in recent years, and more applicants than ever achieve top grades and receive excellent references from their schools. In response to this, admissions tests are now used in certain subjects with the aim of providing an alternative method of assessing a candidate's aptitude, in addition to your exam results and personal statement. These tests are important but are only an alternative method of assessment and should be seen as another way to demonstrate your strengths rather than something to be concerned about!

This list is not exhaustive - UCAS Apply will warn you if additional information such as the above are required, but find out as early as you can so you can prepare.

BTEC STUDENTS
Before applying always check entry requirements carefully, in particular for universities such as Oxford, Cambridge, UCL, Imperial College London and the LSE who may not offer places to students studying BTECs – have a look on the university's website or visit ucas.com for university-specific information.

INDEPENDENT LEARNERS
If you are home-schooled you will be classified as an independent learner and the process is slightly different. When registering you'll need to select the independent option and then complete the UCAS form in the same way, but adding the details of your chosen referee in the reference section. Once you've finished, it allows you to generate an email which will be sent to your referee. Make sure you have contacted them first to ask if this is OK! They will need to

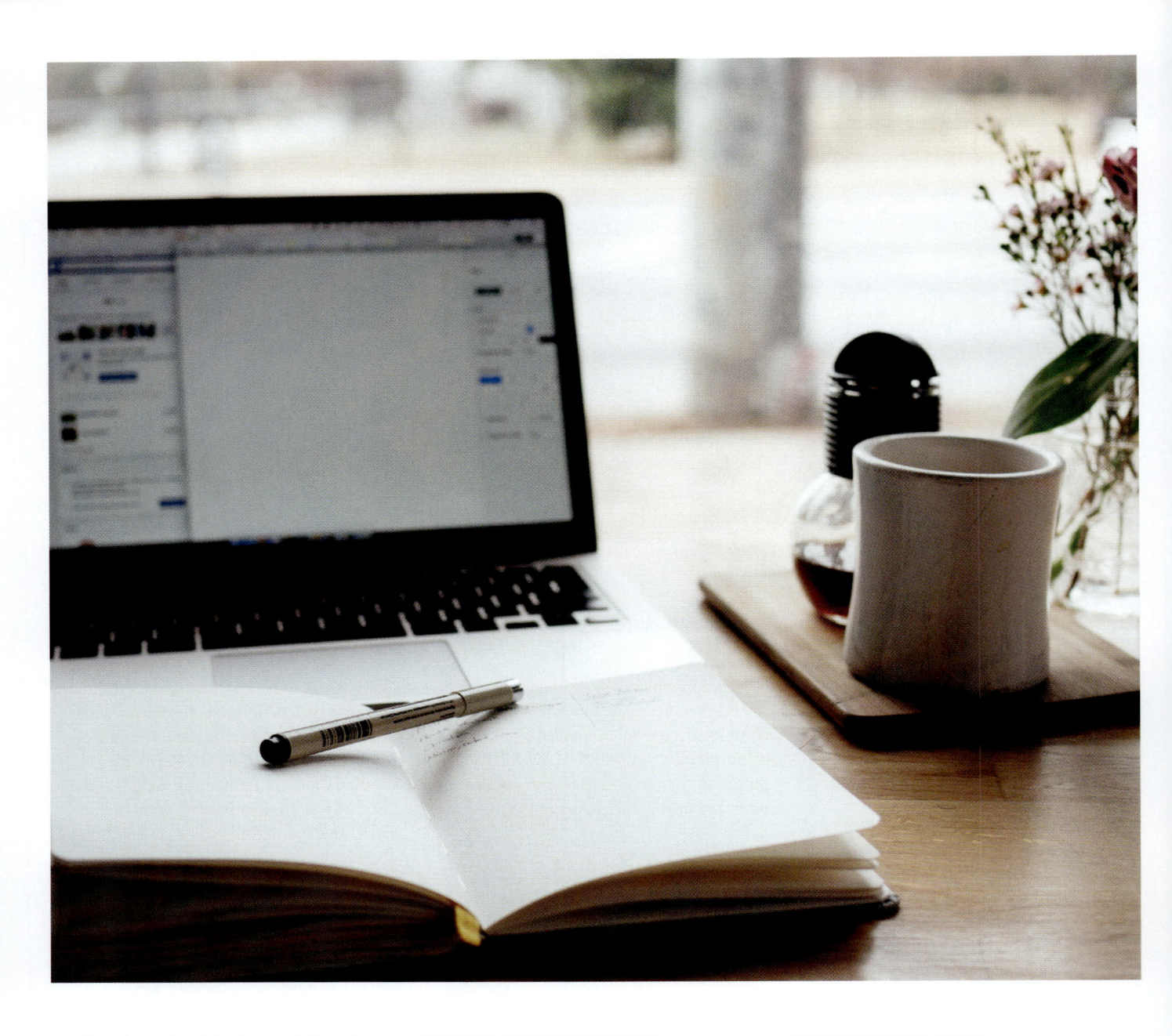

confirm their identification and then give their reference and your predicted grades. It will only be once they complete this that you will be able to pay your fee and submit the application.

What happens next?

Once UCAS has your application you will have to play the nail-biting waiting game. It can take a while for the responses to trickle through because UCAS has to process hundreds of thousands of applications. Also, don't expect them all to come at once – it can be as quick as a week or two, or as long as months.

OFFERS AND REJECTIONS

You will be able to view the status of your application via UCAS Track on their website, and UCAS will email you whenever there is news. When you do finally hear back you will get one of the following:

Offer conditional

A conditional offer means that you must get certain grades on results day in order to be accepted.

Offer unconditional

In rare cases an unconditional offer is given, and it means that whatever you get your place is guaranteed!

Unsuccessful

If you have not been awarded a place you will be sent a notification that your application has been unsuccessful.

FIRM & INSURANCE

You will be asked to pick two offers when you hear from all the unis, and you will choose one 'Firm' and another 'Insurance'. Usually the best thing to do is put your first choice university with the higher grade requirements as your Firm offer, and have a back-up uni that you would still like to attend with lower grade requirements as your Insurance. If you don't get any offers at all you can go through what is known as UCAS Extra.

If you've got your responses and chosen your Firm and Insurance then all that remains is to study hard, and smash those exams.

The UCAS application timeline

Summer 2018
Choose your course and up to 5 universities.
Write the first draft of your personal statement.
Register with UCAS and begin your online application.

1st September 2018
Applications open.
Your school or college will write your reference.

15th October 2018
Admissions deadline for Oxford, Cambridge, medicine, dentistry and veterinary.

October – November 2018
Most admissions tests (double check as UKCAT opens earlier in May).

October 2018 – May 2019
Interviews.
Start to hear back from the universities: conditional, unconditional or unsuccessful.

15th January 2019
Admissions deadline for the majority of courses.

Late February – early July 2019
Extra – chance to add another choice if you've used all five choices and are not holding any offers.

March 2019
Deadline for some art & design courses.

March 2019
Apply for student finance.

May – June 2019
Exams.

Early July – September 2019
Clearing – used if applied after 30th June, didn't receive any offers (or none you wanted to accept) or didn't meet the conditions of your offers.

August 2019
A-Level results day.
Clearing or adjustment.

September 2019
University or gap year begins!

How to handle A-Level results day

It's been a black mark in your calendar all summer and you break out in a cold sweat just by thinking about it. Every sixth form student in the nation will go to bed the night before with a little fear in their hearts, no matter how confident they felt when they walked out of the exam hall, or what they were predicted.

There are several options for Year 13 students on A-Level results day and depending on the grades you get, one of them will apply to you. We strongly recommend reading all of the options before the big day so that you are fully prepared for any outcome.

Your future is not something to make hasty decisions over, so take your time to consider your next step. If you don't meet your expected grades, and you don't think you could improve if you retake, then perhaps you should consider if academia really is for you (if you get higher grades than expected then see Option Five, Adjustment). There are plenty of highly-regarded alternatives to university, so if you think that going straight into employment could be the route for you, have a look at the careers section. There are plenty of programmes which combine studying for qualifications with practical, vocational experience – investigate all the options available and don't have the blinkered and out-dated view that the only route to success is through higher education.

BE HERE

Make sure you have nothing scheduled on the big day so you can go to school first thing to find out your grades. If you do have to be away, ensure you have reliable, fast internet and telephone access! You will need to sign into UCAS Track to see the outcome of your application. UCAS Track will not display your actual grades, but you should be able to get these via your school so ask your teacher before hand.

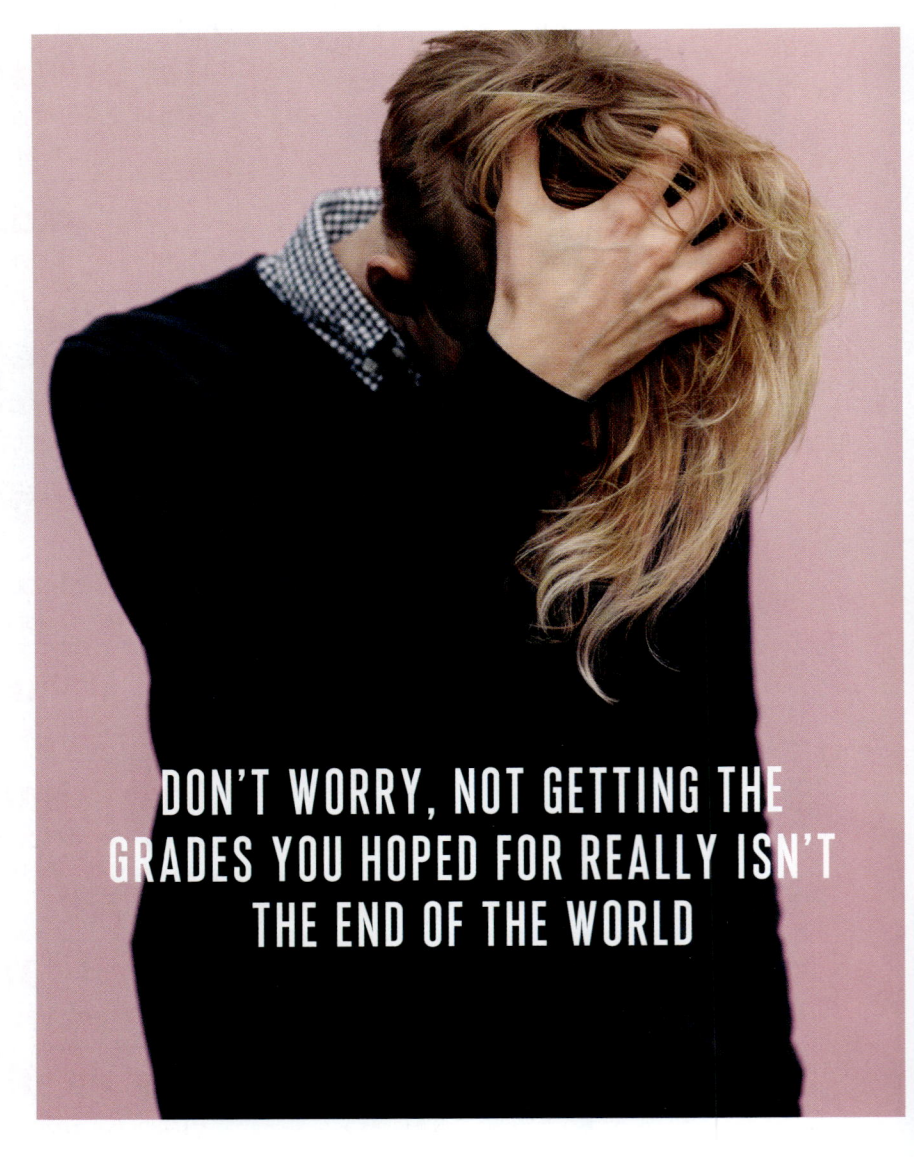

BE PREPARED

However confident you are of meeting your grade requirements, it's always a good idea to research your alternatives in advance. Just as you researched your first choice universities and courses, or school leaver programme or apprenticeship thoroughly, it is important to do the same again using websites and prospectuses, (or even open days if you still have time) so you know what your options are. Having a broad, objective view of what you would consider doing if you missed or exceeded your expected grades will allow you to make an informed and rational decision on the day, should you need to.

It's also important to speak to staff at your school and find out what support they offer on the day, what time they open, who will be there, and if there will be anyone you can talk to.

> **DON'T WORRY, NOT GETTING THE GRADES YOU HOPED FOR REALLY ISN'T THE END OF THE WORLD**

Your 6 options are:

1. Accepting
2. Clearing
3. Remarking
4. Retaking
5. Adjustment
6. Deferring

OPTION ONE: ACCEPTING

If you got the results you were expecting, then well done. If you are still sure that you want to go to university, embark on the school leaver programme or job you've applied for, or head off on your gap year then that's fantastic! Or, if you haven't made any plans yet but you're pleased with your results then you can get on with thinking about what you'd like to do next, safe in the knowledge that you got the grades you wanted.

PLEASE NOTE:

If you change your mind about what you want to do then make sure you let the relevant people know. You never know when your paths may cross again in the future, so it is important to thank them for the opportunity, and briefly explain your reasons for withdrawing. They will understand.

OPTION TWO: CLEARING

If you get poorer-than-expected exam results but these are just a blip in an otherwise good academic performance to date and you still want to go to uni, then Clearing could be for you. Don't worry, not getting the grades you hoped for really isn't the end of the world, even though it might feel that way at first. Last year over 45,000 students secured a place at university through Clearing so don't be disheartened. The rule of thumb here is not to jump the gun and go with the first half-decent offer you get!

YOU ARE ELIGIBLE FOR CLEARING IF...

· You have not received any offers

· You have declined all your offers or not responded by the due date

· Your offers have not been confirmed because you have not met the conditions (e.g. you have not achieved the required grades)

· You applied for one course which has been declined / unsuccessful and you have paid the full £24 fee (if you only applied to one university through 'single choice' then you will need to pay the full fee of £24 to enter Clearing)

· UCAS receive your application after 30th June deadline (if they receive your application after this date, UCAS will not send it to any universities and colleges)

MIDNIGHT - VACANCIES PUBLISHED

All vacancies will be published on the UCAS website just after midnight the day of A-Level results day. Most students don't get much sleep that night anyway so it's worth staying up to have a thorough scroll through this list and pick out any courses or universities that might be of interest.

Many leading universities offer well-respected courses through Clearing, so don't be under the impression that it's only the dregs left!

PLEASE NOTE:

It is possible that if you only just missed your grades by a few marks, your chosen university might still offer you a place, so contact them as soon as you can.

CLEARING CONTINUED:

Call the institutions you are interested in and talk to them about your situation, they will be sympathetic! You can find out which ones have vacancies on the UCAS website. You will need to give them your Clearing number and UCAS Personal ID number which will allow them to see your original application online.

We recommend having a reasonable explanation ready for missing your grades, and other credentials such as your mock exam results, as well as a copy of your personal statement printed and to hand so you can refer to it easily. If you change your mind about the type of degree you intend to study then expect that the institution may want to know why - you'll have to be convincing because they will want you to demonstrate commitment!

Get a few informal offers from universities covering all the areas of interest, at institutions you can genuinely see yourself going to. Have a browse through their websites, and read more about what their specific course entails. Don't be disheartened if a few universities reject you, and certainly don't give up. You have the whole day to choose what to do, because UCAS won't accept Clearing entries until 5pm. We can't stress the importance of taking your time over this decision. Talk to teachers, friends, relatives, careers advisors… but most importantly ask yourself the pros and cons of your options.

5PM: ENTER YOUR CLEARING CHOICE

By entering a choice through Clearing you are accepting the offer, so only do this when the final decision is made. If the course is still available then you will be notified, and then you will receive a letter in the post shortly after to confirm your place. If the places are full then you will be allowed to add another option, so wait until you have been accepted before leaving the computer screen!

OPTION THREE: REMARKING

You should find out from your school who the designated Examinations Officer is, and if they will be present on the day in case you want a remark. If they won't be there, find out their name, email and phone number in case you want to appeal. If your grade is much lower than you had expected, the Examinations Officer can ask the exam board to send your paper to be remarked. This could be particularly important if you have fallen on a grade boundary and it could make the difference between getting into university or not.

Exam boards must receive your request (made on your behalf by your school) by the end of August. It is possible to ask for a priority remark. This applies if it is a matter of missing your existing university offer and your university will be able to hold your offer until you hear the results. It is important to be aware that there is a charge for remarking A-Level papers. This is sometimes paid for by your school, but you must check this. If your grade changes you will, of course, be refunded.

Each exam board has different remark options available, so you must check the relevant website to find out what your exam board's policies are. Most commonly, you will be offered a clerical check, which verifies whether your grade was calculated and entered onto the system properly. If your teacher has concerns about several students' examination results, the exam board might well offer to remark 10% of the papers from your class. If, as a result of this check, several pupils are given higher grades, this could positively affect the rest of the class' marks.

PLEASE NOTE

The most important thing to remember is that your mark could also go down as well as up, so the process is a risky one. You should talk to your teacher to see whether he or she thinks that remarking is the right option for you.

OPTION FOUR: RETAKING

It is also possible to re-sit your examinations in June the following year; the January re-sit option is no longer available. While this will involve a great deal of extra work, revision and taking a gap year, it could be less risky than asking for your papers to be remarked because if you happen to do worse in your re-sits, you can keep your original grade.

Speak to your school about what they offer if you want to retake. You may also need to attend a different sixth form or FE college in the local area to do this. This option is particularly useful if, for any reason, you didn't have the chance to revise as much as you could have, or if there were any distracting circumstances at home which might have affected your exams.

PLEASE NOTE

You need to be sure that with extra hard work you can do significantly better – you may have to defer entry to university so be sure that the extra time and commitment is likely to pay off.

OPTION FIVE: ADJUSTMENT

If you have done better in your A-Levels than you expected, congratulations! It is possible for you to apply for another university without losing your secure offer.

UCAS Adjustment allows students with better-than-expected results to effectively 'upgrade' their course and university.

HOW DOES IT WORK?
From the moment that your offer is confirmed by your first choice university, you have five days to try to secure an offer from another university. You will be able to see exactly when your individual Adjustment period ends on the Track 'Choices' page on UCAS.

When you get your results, a 'Register for Adjustment' button will appear on your UCAS Track page. Registering will allow the universities which you decide to contact in the hope of a better offer to look at your whole application. In order to find out which universities are offering places through Adjustment, you need to visit their individual websites where they will list the courses they still have places for. If you are feeling confident about your exam performance, then it's worth doing some research in advance so you know who to target.

Once you shortlist suitable courses, you need to phone up the admissions department of those universities and discuss your application. You might have a short interview on the phone, in which case you will have to explain why you want to take this particular course and what it is about the university that has attracted you to contact them. Don't be put off by this process! The interview will be informal, but make sure you've got a copy of your personal statement close by to refer to. Just be passionate about the course and confident in your results, don't let them think it was a fluke – you got the grades because you deserve them and you worked hard!

If the university or college decides to give you an offer, they will phone you or send you an email, so ensure you have access to both of these throughout the next few days. Once you hear from them keep checking your UCAS Track page so you can accept the offer when it comes through. Once you click accept then your original offer will be affected, so make sure you've thought it through carefully and discussed the decision with teachers and family at length.

The best thing about the Adjustment process is that you can shop around at other universities without losing the offer you have already accepted at your first choice university. Adjustment is becoming a very successful system – in 2014, 1,200 students successfully found a place on a course they considered to be more suitable for them such as Exeter, Durham, Warwick, Birmingham, Sheffield, UCL and King's College London.

THINGS TO KNOW
The Adjustment period only lasts five days, so you have a very short space of time to make a decision. If you do find yourself in this situation, it might be a good idea to speak to a teacher about your options, particularly if you are thinking of changing your course. UCAS and the careers service within each university will have trained advisors who will be available to help you.

Because you will be accepting a new university offer at such a late stage in the year, you might be at the back of the queue for student accommodation, and student finance might be affected too. It would be good to discuss accommodation and finance issues when you phone up the admissions department of the university you wish to apply to.

It is important not to make a spur of the moment decision. If you are happy with the course and university you originally chose, stick with it! Investigate the course content, a course with the same name could have a different structure, different assessment methods and cover completely different topics to your original course.

PLEASE NOTE
You may not be successful. You will not be judged on grades alone, your whole UCAS application will be taken into consideration, and you'll be up against competition from other students going through the process, so it isn't a guarantee.

OPTION SIX: DEFERRING

If, in between submitting your university application and receiving your results, you decide to take a gap year, you should contact the university that you have been accepted into on Results Day and check if you can defer your place for a year.

Explain to the university your reasons for deferring, such as a desire to travel, gain work experience, or become more independent.

PLEASE NOTE
Universities are not obliged to agree to this, but most do. If your university won't allow you to defer, but you have your heart set on a year off, then you still have the option of withdrawing from UCAS and reapplying the following year.

masterclass

Your personal statement is an important part of your application and you need to do everything it takes to get it just right. You have a minimum of 1,000 and a maximum of 4,000 characters (including spaces) to show admissions tutors why they should pick you over other candidates.

Apart from your teacher reference this is the only section of the UCAS form where you will have a chance to show the 'real' you, the person beyond the grades. Don't listen to anyone who says universities don't look at personal statements anymore, because they do. Apart from the main, first round of applications, they can be particularly useful in borderline cases if you're up against another candidate, or if you go through Clearing, so you need to give it your all.

You will need to have decided what you want to study before you start, as the main reason for writing the statement is to prove your suitability and passion for that subject, so if you're still undecided, research how to choose your course first. You'll also need to have looked at the course structure at each and every one of the universities you intend to apply to as there can be significant variations between each course, and get a feel for what they offer, and what they are looking for - and keep this in mind when writing your statement.

We have canvassed many admissions tutors to find out what they are looking for and the result is this masterclass on how to plan and write an outstanding personal statement. Don't forget that tutors will be reading a very large volume of personal statements and you need to make your application stand out from the rest. Assume that the reader is an academic who has devoted his or her life to their chosen subject.

What they really want to know is, have you chosen the right subject for the right reason?

HOW IT WORKS

The Pure Potential Personal Statement Masterclass will help you to write your statement if you follow it step by step and start by writing down as much as you possibly can. Your first few drafts are bound to be rubbish, it's the same for everyone! But it's much easier to cut down on material then it is to come up with it, so jot down everything you can think of in the boxes in bullet points as we go along, we'll edit it down later and turn the best bits into beautiful prose.

If you get stuck on any section then please just move on as you can always come back to it, and we know there's nothing worse than having a mental block or getting stuck in a personal statement rut!

STRUCTURE
There are lots of ways to structure your statement, but Pure Potential's suggestion is approximately 75% dedicated to academic study:

INTRODUCTION
Explain your motivation for studying the subject.

IN-SCHOOL EVIDENCE OF SKILLS & INTEREST (optional)
Briefly mention any specific skills you are learning at school that will be relevant for your course.

EVIDENCE OF YOUR PASSION FOR THE SUBJECT
This must be outside of school so they can see it's a genuine interest!

GAP YEAR PLANS
If applicable.

WIDER SKILLS
What are you doing in or out of school that shows you are a mature, well-rounded person?

CONCLUSION
Remind them why they should pick you.

WRITING YOUR INTRODUCTION

You will need to provide a brief but convincing explanation as to why you want to study your subject at university. This should capture the reader's interest straight away so they are compelled to read on. Here are some suggestions of how to start your statement, but please don't use all of the suggestions below – choose one or two that are right for you, or come up with your own:

YOUR PERSONAL TRIGGER

What got you interested in the subject? Was it a book, a museum trip, a documentary, a film, a teacher, an inspirational mentor, a personal circumstance, a visit to a historical site, or perhaps work experience? Don't ever say 'I have always been interested in "INSERT SUBJECT"'! This is a cliché that admissions tutors are sick of reading, because it can't possibly be true! Nobody was born with a desire to be a doctor, lawyer or engineer. For example, an applicant might explain how their family holiday to the Somme gave them a genuine sense of the importance of history as a 'real life' phenomenon - something that exists beyond the pages of a textbook.

THE BIG PICTURE

Why is this subject important? Is it significant to the progression of society? What about our understanding of natural history and evolution? Will your subject lead to the betterment of lives of future generations? Does it shape the world we live in somehow? What's going on in the world right now that relates to your subject? This could be anything from cutting-edge scientific research or technology, grey areas in morality or justice, the state of the world's economy, or how looking at ancient civilisations or different cultures helps us to understand who we are. Why do you want to be part of the academic community researching this subject further?

SPECIFIC AREAS OF INTEREST

Having given a broad account of why you love your subject, focus on specific areas of interest within it. For example, if you want to study physics, you could go on to say how it's really the module on astrophysics that gets your pulse racing, and in what way you hope the degree course will develop your passion further. You will need to read the course prospectus for all the universities you are applying to before you write this!

USING QUOTES

We often get asked by students if it is a good idea to start the statement with a fancy quote from an expert in the field, famous author or scientist. Almost every admissions tutor we have spoken to would rather you didn't use one! It is only acceptable to do this if you directly relate it to your course and why you want to study it, show that you fully understand the concept of the quote and use it to enhance your own words instead of just using somebody else's but if you can say it in your own words then do so.

CAREER PLANS

If you have a definite or even a rough idea of what you want to do when you graduate, and your university degree is a stepping stone towards that aspiration then you may wish to write it here. If you have no idea don't worry, many people don't. If you're a budding medic, dentist or similar then you will need to go into further depth, but for all others remember that you are applying for an academic degree, not a job so don't focus too much on your career.

FILL IN THE BOXES RELEVANT TO YOU:

WHAT WAS MY PERSONAL TRIGGER?

_____

HOW DOES MY SUBJECT RELATE TO SOCIETY OR CURRENT AFFAIRS? WHY IS THIS PARTICULARLY IMPORTANT TO ME?

_____

WHICH ASPECT AM I REALLY LOOKING FORWARD TO STUDYING IN MORE DETAIL? WHY?

_____

IS THERE A QUOTE I LIKE THE SOUND OF? COULD I EXPRESS THIS IN MY OWN WORDS?

_____

WHAT ARE MY CAREER PLANS? HOW MIGHT ACADEMIC STUDY FURTHER MY PLANS?

_____

IN-SCHOOL EVIDENCE OF SKILLS & INTERESTS (optional)

WHY OPTIONAL?
This section is optional because you should only talk about current studies if you can talk about them impressively and academically. Not everyone will be able to, or should, relate their current studies to their chosen course, and in fact this section pales in significance to evidence of what you've done out of school, so don't worry if you leave it blank!

Don't forget that every one of your fellow candidates (aka your competition) is studying A-Levels, BTECS, IBs or equivalent, so school work is not going to make you stand out, unless you can truly demonstrate your understanding of how your current studies can specifically help your chosen degree course.

WHAT NOT TO DO
What they DON'T want to see is something like this, 'I currently study Maths, English and Biology at A-Level. Maths helps with my problem-solving skills, English helps with essay writing, and Biology has given me an understanding of human anatomy'. Firstly, they know what you study at A-Level from the rest of your application form, so don't waste precious words on repeating this information. Secondly, these examples linking your current studies to your degree course are hardly insightful. Far better examples of skills you have picked up during your school studies are critical analysis of evidence, laboratory work or the ability to study independently. Thirdly, don't feel you have to mention each and every one of your subjects, if you pick any, just pick the relevant ones.

SPRINGBOARD
We also suggest that you tell them how your current studies have been a springboard for further reading in your own time. If you take on further independent reading on a topic that interests you, and show enthusiasm for seeing how theories you learn apply to the real world, then you are exactly the type of student universities are looking for. It's not too late either – a quick Google in your chosen area will open up a whole world of related topics for you to mention. Name drop what you read, who wrote it and what was interesting, this leads nicely into the next paragraph.

A-LEVEL / BTEC / IB / etc	RELEVANT SKILLS DEVELOPED
SUBJECT 1	
SUBJECT 2	
SUBJECT 3	
SUBJECT 4	
SUBJECT 5	
SUBJECT 6	
SUBJECT 7	
SUBJECT 8	

EVIDENCE OF YOUR PASSION FOR THE SUBJECT

This is by far the most important part of your statement where you can really shine because it's the things you've done in your own time which will show a genuine passion for the subject. Remember that one of the main differences between university and school is that there's no one looking over your shoulder, making sure you do your homework. You have to show that you are self-motivated to do things outside of the classroom or lecture theatre. For most students these activities will come under the categories below. Tick all that apply to you and, crucially, are specifically relevant to the course you have chosen. First write down a list of things you've done, then write down what you learnt from that experience / book / documentary / trip that will directly help your degree course. Make sure you name all authors, directors, places, companies, books etc. We've given you a list of suggestions for each category, but don't worry, you're only expected to have done a few from each list!

You may end up with up to three paragraphs for this section – that's OK!

WIDER READING

One excellent way of demonstrating passion is through wider reading, and admissions tutors are looking for students who are willing to read around the subject in their own time. "But I don't know what to read?" we hear you ask! One of the best places to look for reading lists is on the university website. They usually have a list of suggested books for undergraduates, most of which will be available in your local library. If you can't find a reading list, then speak to your teachers, or even call the department of the university you want to apply for – they'll be more than happy to recommend a book or two!

	DETAILS	WHAT DID YOU LEARN?
Textbooks		
Plays		
Poetry		
Passages		
Articles		
Journals		
Newspapers		
Other		

OTHER RESEARCH

There are more interactive ways of researching your chosen subject that will convince admission tutors you are truly interested. Many of these can be free of charge.

	DETAILS	WHAT DID YOU LEARN?
Theatre trips		
Art exhibitions		
Museum trips		
Historical sites		
Geographical landmarks		
Film documentaries		
Podcasts eg. Ted		
Other		

RELEVANT WORK EXPERIENCE

If you've undertaken any work experience which relates to your subject then write it down here (save the casual weekend jobs for the next section). Did hands-on work reinforce any principles you have only learnt in theory, such as the importance of accuracy, trustworthiness, efficiency, collaboration, empathy, or any number of things that show how you deepened your understanding of the subject. We're NOT looking for generic skills like time-management and general communication here. And don't forget to name drop the companies.

	DETAILS	WHAT DID YOU LEARN?
Voluntary work		
Work experience		
Paid employment		
Internships		
Community activities		
Other		
Other		

COURSE-RELATED PROGRAMMES

Many universities and other organisations offer you the chance to sample your chosen subject through taster opportunities. These tend to get fully booked quickly, so find out what's going on and where, as early on as possible. We advise a scattergun approach – apply to lots of programmes; you'll learn a lot even if they are at a university you don't intend to apply to.

	DETAILS	WHAT DID YOU LEARN?
Webinars		
Workshops		
Laboratory work		
Lectures		
Masterclasses		
Residentials		
Summer school		
Other		
Other		

OTHER ACTIVITIES

What else have you done that shows you're interested in the subject?

	DETAILS	WHAT DID YOU LEARN?
Competitions		
Prizes		
Awards		
Published work		
Hobbies		
Collections		
Other		

GAP YEAR PLANS

If you are taking a gap year and applying for deferred entry then you should explain what you plan to do briefly in this section – give details and don't be ashamed of backpacking with friends around some far-flung land. Telling the admissions tutor about your plans for the year ahead shows that you are organised, and want to pursue interests outside of your studies, which is healthy and makes you a well-rounded person. If you can relate it to the course, or university life, that's even better. It is an academic application, so don't bang on about this too much, even if you're secretly more excited about travelling than starting university!

Plans for my gap year:

How will I fund them?

What am I hoping to achieve or get out of the experience?

How will this help me with my degree, university life or career?

WIDER SKILLS

This is where you will give an account of your non-academic achievements and the skills you picked up along the way through your interests and hobbies either in or out of school. Cover any extra-curricular activities not necessarily related to your course to give the admissions tutor a glimpse of the kind of person you are outside of the classroom.

The table below has a list of skills you may have developed. Alongside each skill enter the most relevant activity – try to pick just one activity per skill, even if you learnt more than one skill from it. Here are some examples: if you have volunteered as a reading mentor for younger students, this would definitely have developed your communication skills; you developed an efficient approach to solving problems during your work experience and you also showed great initiative; if you're on the football team you would have developed team working skills; a prefect might have a sense of responsibility; living abroad will make you more adaptable; directing a play would give you leadership skills etc. etc. etc.

What kind of things have you done? Sports, school plays, volunteering, fundraising, organising events, community work, a part-time job, other hobbies – this list will be endless because you're all doing such diverse things…

Remember to make yourself stand out. Juggling a Saturday job with studies isn't going to achieve that because thousands of sixth formers do it. You need to demonstrate you've gone the extra mile.

In the box below, fill in the top one or two skills you learnt along the way, here are some examples:

	DETAILS	WHAT DID YOU LEARN?
Communication		
Commitment		
Time management		
Teamwork		
Using initiative		
Public speaking		
Adaptability		
Organisation		
Leadership		
Research & analysis		
Maturity		
Responsibility		
Other		

CONCLUSION

People often struggle with this, but it should be an easy paragraph once you've written the rest. Simply finish the personal statement with a one or two line summary of why you are a suitable candidate, what you hope to get out of, and give to, the university community. Make sure this sentence convinces the tutor of how much you're looking forward to it all, so use really aspirational language!

EXAMPLES

"Overall, I am a hardworking, active person and I am enthusiastic about achieving my goals and becoming a primary school teacher. I am looking forward to university life, both academically and socially."

"I am mature, confident and self-motivated - all qualities that I believe are critical to a successful university experience. I relish the opportunity to study Accountancy and Finance to degree level and hopefully beyond."

"I feel certain that this subject will provide me with the intellectual challenge best suited to my personality and ambition of pursuing an academic career in the social sciences. The prospect of studying a stimulating and dynamic course truly excites me."

WRITE YOUR OWN

_____

_____

_____

_____

_____

_____

YOUR FIRST DRAFT

Look back at the tables you've filled in – it might not look like it at the moment but this is your first draft! The next step is to choose which points are the most important ones to include.

So what are the admissions tutors looking for? Well, first and foremost it is the things you have done that show passion for the course; the more 'outside of school' evidence the better. Skills such as time management and teamwork are great, but are secondary to evidence of a desire to study a subject. If you can 'double up' on skills and talk about things you have learnt and what you have done to demonstrate your interest in the subject at the same time as one of these skills, then great!

For example, you did work experience at your local medical centre and learnt the importance of patient confidentiality, as well as developing an interest in a health-related career. You may well have also developed excellent communication skills by answering the telephone, contributing to meetings, and interacting with staff and patients.

Go back and look at all that you wrote down, and highlight, or circle the aspects that you think an admissions tutor will find most impressive, and re-write them as brief bullet points in the space opposite:

Introduction

In-school evidence of skills & interest (optional)

Evidence of your passion for the subject

Wider skills

Conclusion

TURNING IT INTO PROSE

We can't teach you how to write well, but we can give you examples of positive phrases and key words that can help you link sentences together, and combine your experiences with skills. Choose some of these positive phrases and start putting sentences together, crossing each phrase off as you go along to avoid repetition. Add some phrases of your own too for originality.

FINAL NOTES

- Transfer the activities you have deemed worthy of your personal statement to a Word document. If in doubt, include it, because you can always edit it out later. Don't worry about going over the word count at this stage. And don't forget to save regularly!

- Many people find it easier to work on the introduction last. It doesn't matter which order you do it in, as long as you end up with the same structure – subheadings can work well here to maintain order, but don't include this in your final statement. Choose the activity or topic you feel most comfortable talking about first to get the flow of writing started.

- Give enough detail, but don't bore them; 2-3 sentences on any topic should be enough.

- Illustrate your skills and abilities rather than state them, nothing worse than ending a good sentence with 'and this shows I have communication skills'.

- Do not state facts about the subject such as, 'Geography is the subject that studies the lands, the features, the inhabitants, and the phenomena of the Earth'.

- Do not say lofty, important-sounding things you cannot back up, for example, 'The complexity of life and the Universe itself shows that the human race has only scratched the surface of knowledge'.

- Do not use negative words like never, hate, useless, mistake, tiring, stressful etc.

- Personal statement advice can seem conflicting: be yourself but don't use humour, demonstrate a good vocabulary but don't overuse the thesaurus, be confident but not cocky, show your passion but don't use the word passion, show your skills but don't list them! We know it is hard, but try to find a balance once you get to the proofreading stage.

- Furthermore
- Enable me
- Of particular interest to me
- On reflection
- Intellectual exploration
- Additionally
- Used my initiative
- Strengthen
- Explore my interests
- Skills I have gained through
- Thrive under pressure
- As well as
- Commitment
- Reinforced
- This has furthered my
- I learned from
- Moreover
- My pursuits
- Taking part in
- Creatively
- Benefit
- Efficiently
- In addition
- Hard work
- I undertook
- I aspire to
- My interest in
- Responsibility
- I particularly enjoyed
- I continue to develop
- Through regularly attending
- To improve my
- Combining... with... has taught me
- This has expanded my knowledge o
- Challenging
- Immensely rewarding
- Brought to my attention
- Thought-provoking
- Learnt to prioritise
- Highly competitive

PROOFREADING

Checking and editing your personal statement should take up as much time as creating the first draft, so don't leave it to the last minute. In fact, you can reasonably expect to have over 20 drafts before you have a submission-ready version. If you have time, we suggest leaving it for a few days to clear your head. Then read it again. Every single line should be a new reason for the admissions tutor to pick you:

· Be ruthless! Get rid of any repetition or waffle.

· Don't have any 'don't's or 'I'll's or 'I'm's! This is a formal document.

· Spelling and grammar must be perfect! NO EXCUSES.

· Don't TRY and sound clever! You are clever and this will shine through, have faith in your achievements.

· Be careful with capitals! Make sure you are correct, and consistent.

· Then ask parents, friends, friends of your parents, employers, mentors – literally anyone you can think of to check through your statement.

· Do your best to get rid of typos before asking people to look at it so they can focus on the content and not silly grammatical errors.

· Don't send it out to everyone all at once, otherwise you'll get lots of different versions back which can be overwhelming. Send it to one person, get their feedback, apply the feedback, then send it on again.

· Don't be surprised if you get conflicting advice from different people – sometimes there is no right or wrong, so if this happens go with your gut instinct.

· Be sure to say please and thank you – so many people forget to ask nicely and show their appreciation!

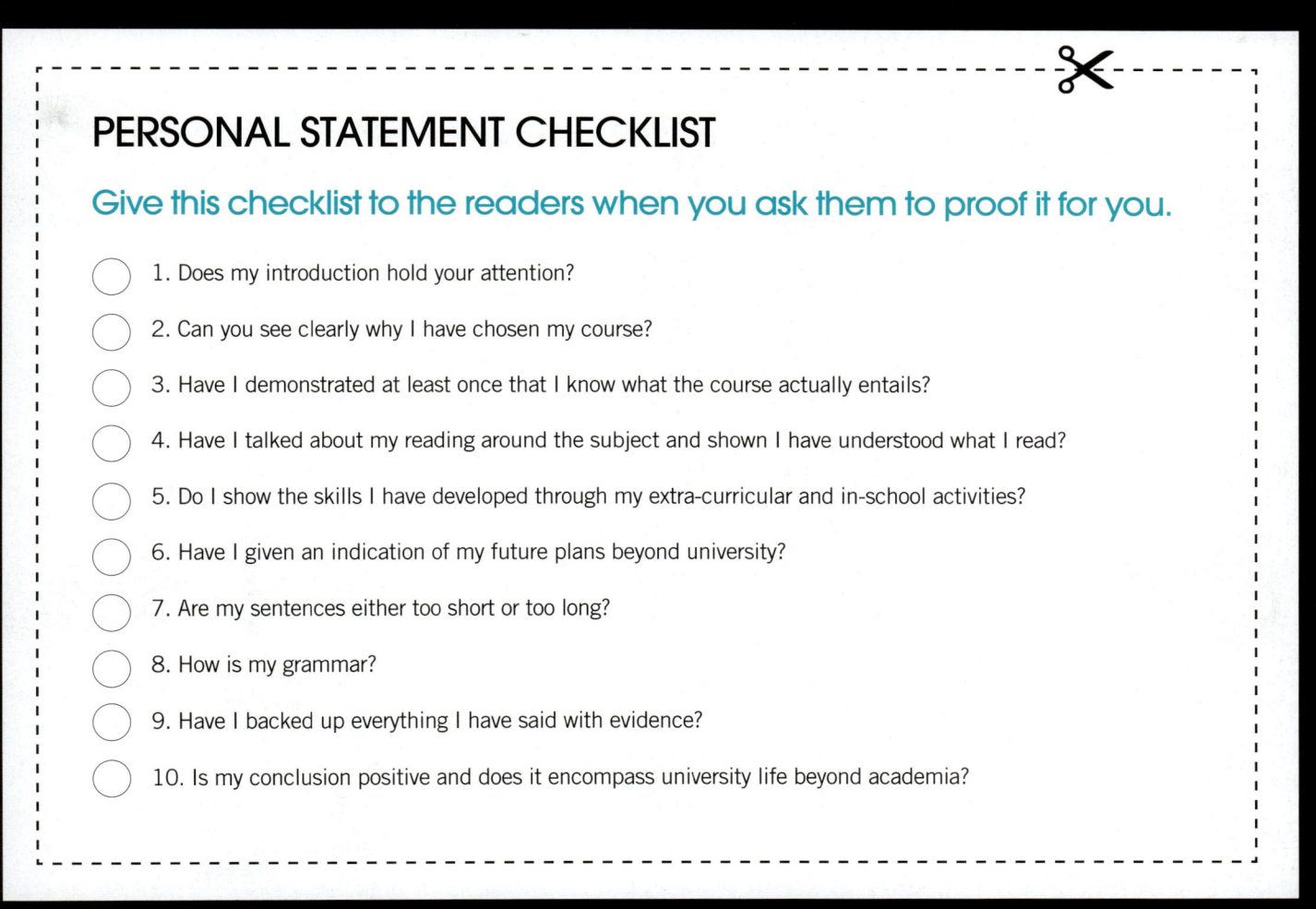

PERSONAL STATEMENT CHECKLIST

Give this checklist to the readers when you ask them to proof it for you.

- ◯ 1. Does my introduction hold your attention?
- ◯ 2. Can you see clearly why I have chosen my course?
- ◯ 3. Have I demonstrated at least once that I know what the course actually entails?
- ◯ 4. Have I talked about my reading around the subject and shown I have understood what I read?
- ◯ 5. Do I show the skills I have developed through my extra-curricular and in-school activities?
- ◯ 6. Have I given an indication of my future plans beyond university?
- ◯ 7. Are my sentences either too short or too long?
- ◯ 8. How is my grammar?
- ◯ 9. Have I backed up everything I have said with evidence?
- ◯ 10. Is my conclusion positive and does it encompass university life beyond academia?

FINALLY, RUN IT BY YOUR TEACHER

Listen carefully to their advice - they go through this process every year and can draw on valuable experience. Make sure you give them plenty of time to give it proper attention, not 5 minutes before the school deadline!

EXAMPLE PERSONAL STATEMENT

Here is a model personal statement for the fictional subject of comedy studies:

I believe that laughter is fundamental to human experience. Basil Fawlty, John Cleese's comic creation in 'Fawlty Towers', once said, 'Still, you've got to laugh, haven't you?'. We have to laugh because, far from being a distraction or mere entertainment, comedy represents our attempt to reconcile ourselves to some of the deepest human truths, like death and love. I want to study this course to further my understanding both of the history and evolution of comedy, and to improve my critical skills so that I can unravel the whole meaning of each joke and scene.

[Here the student clearly explains what inspires him to study the course. He included a quote, but it is short, embedded in the text, and its meaning is clearly explained. He also demonstrates he understands what the course entails, and expresses enthusiasm]

Comedy Studies A-Level has opened my eyes the potential of comedy to create social change: we studied, 'Bremner, Bird and Fortune, which opened my eyes to politics and the hypocrisies of government in a way conventional news never could. Theoretical study of political satire has led me to research this further in my own time by watching current and historical television shows such as 'Spitting Image, 'Have I got News for You' and 'Mock the Week'. I set myself the task of writing my own show, 'Politically Correct?' which was turned into a school play that I also directed.

[The student discusses his current studies, but briefly and using an insightful example of what he has learnt. He goes on to use this as a springboard to talk about independent study, name-dropping the shows he watched and throws in his achievement of directing a play too]

Having studied the television show 'The Office' in my own time, I became interested in the idea that the conventional sitcom is dead, and documentary realism is the future of televised comedy. To further my understanding of cultural and national differences in humour, I watched the American version of the same show. I found there to be significant changes to the script, for example, the famous cringe-worthy scene in the British version where David Brent dances has been completely rewritten for American audiences; perhaps different use of sarcasm between the two countries means that the timing of punch lines must be adapted.

I completed work experience helping to write scripts for television shows 'People Like Us' and 'Human Remains'. These two series chart the development of this comic genre, which, unlike the older cheerful sitcoms, deliberately confronts the depths of human despair and failure. Seeing the difference between a line that seemed funny on paper and how it was delivered by the actors on-set showed me how objective comedy can be, and the challenges that face script-writers. To obtain an alternative point of view I also booked tickets to see Channel 4's comedy, 'The Graham Norton Show', being filmed live in London. The experience showed me that comedy can have a vital and performative quality when filmed in front of a live studio audience, and the differences between scripted and off-the-cuff humour.

I have been a regular television reviewer for the local magazine, 'The Pieshop'. Writing reviews has helped me to hone my critical style, and to appraise programmes in a lively and concise way. I also took on the challenge of playing Caliban in the school play of 'The Tempest', an experience which helped me to gain an insight into comedy from the performer's point of view as well as develop my confidence immensely. I also founded the comedy club at school, we have weekly meetings to discuss programmes, I enjoy having heated debates with my peers on what they find funny.

[He has divided his out-of-school experiences into three neat paragraphs that illustrate a broad understanding of various elements of comedy. He talks about what he learnt in a way that shows he is genuinely interested in the subject and engaged with each experience. He has clearly done a range of experience so his third paragraph covers a few experiences in less detail]

I am in the school football team, I enjoy the regular team meetings to improve our performance, and it was immensely rewarding when we won the county cup. I also mentor students at a local primary school and teach them to read. I also ran for, and was elected, the Head Boy position on the Sixth Form Student Council. We regularly liaise with the Upper School students on a range of non-academic issues, and present our findings to the School Governors monthly. These roles have taught me how to balance my studies and extra-curricular responsibilities, which is important because I hope to continue both my sporting and voluntary activities while at university.

[This paragraph is brief but paints a picture of the type of person he is. Also, teamwork, leadership and time management are included in this paragraph without stating them]

Comedy is something I have come back to, inside and outside of the classroom, throughout my life. I think I have the intellectual curiosity, the ability and, most importantly, the sense of humour to gain a much deeper understanding of this subject at university, and would love the opportunity to do so.

[Brief, enthusiastic, positive and a summary of why they should pick him]

USEFUL RESOURCE   purepotential.org - Read over 100 past personal statements annotated by the Pure Potential team.

Enrichment

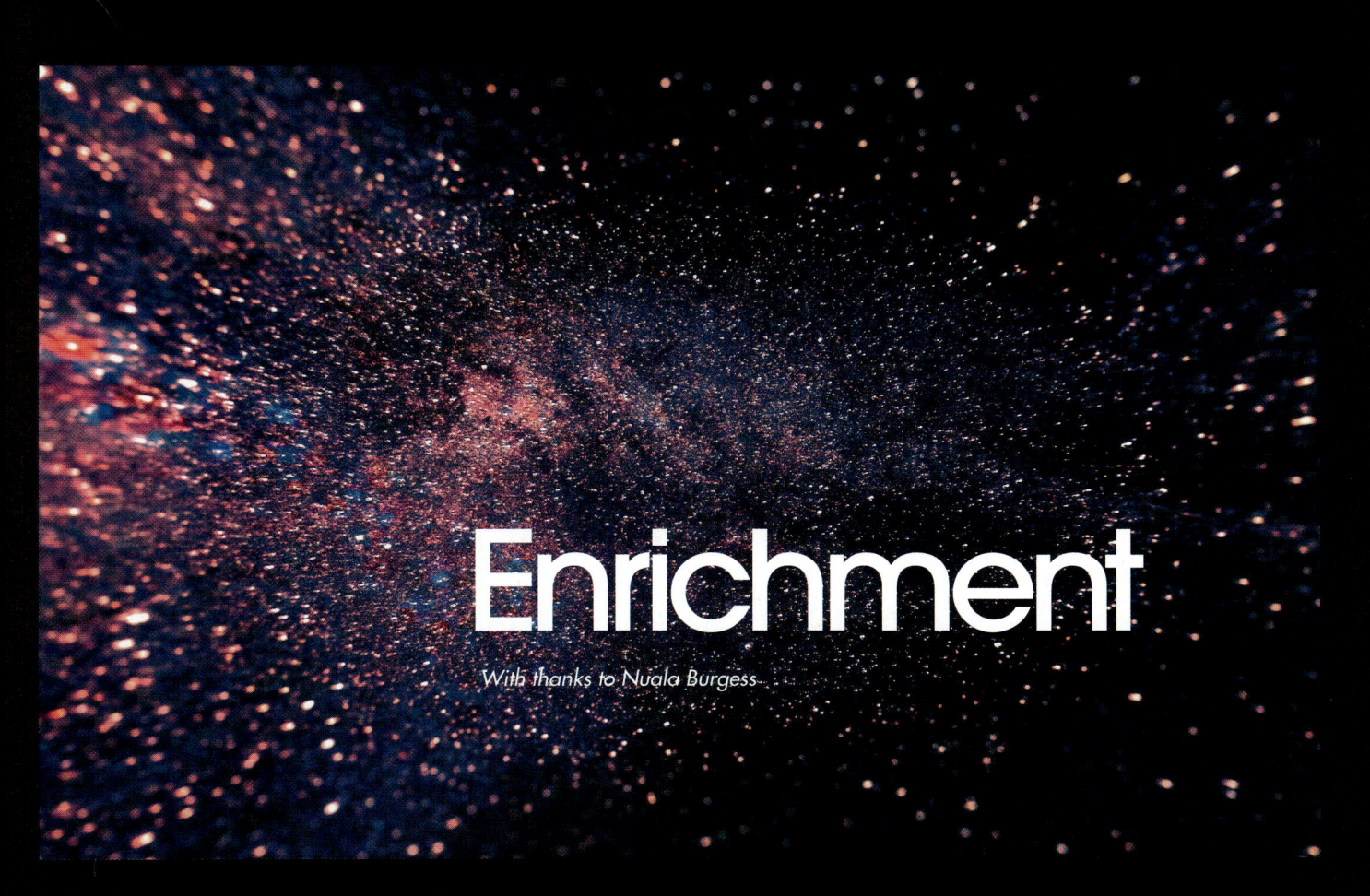

With thanks to Nuala Burgess

Everyone can write a personal statement that sparkles - it's just a matter of knowing how. Whether you are a scientist, a linguist, a student of the humanities, a mathematician or a potential lawyer or medic, the trick is to think creatively about ways to enrich your personal statement.

Our most prestigious universities are looking for intellectual curiosity that goes beyond A-Level subjects.

It is especially impressive if you have discovered an author, or followed a political commentator or a science journalist, or kept up to date with a significant court case in the news, and become a 'specialist' in something that you have made your own. Perhaps you have discovered the social commentary contained in Willkie Collins' Victorian novels or in the slick American detective novels of Raymond Chandler? Perhaps in reading the legal arguments of a significant court case in the news you have begun to question whether law and justice are the same thing? Do you feel particularly strongly about environmental or human rights issues - why? Are you an historian interested in how past revolutions shed light on contemporary social upheavals? Perhaps you are a potential medic with something to say about the ethics of animal testing? Are languages where you shine? Do you relish the challenge of translating the sensibilities of Pablo Neruda's love poetry into English, or are you someone who has discovered the power of Italian neo-realist film or French cinema verité? Whatever it is, find a specialist area of cultural interest and be an expert in your chosen field.

Aim for something that no-one else will be discussing in their personal statement to make yours the most interesting the admissions tutor will read.

If you can't think where to start, try a Saturday or Sunday newspaper - ideally, a paper with a good reputation for its journalism. Both The Guardian and the Daily Telegraph have recently won awards for their investigative and political journalism and both papers contain excellent reviews of literature, art, theatre and film. Skim read your chosen paper and notice which sections really interest you. Avoiding football scores and celebrity gossip, which headlines grabbed your attention? Was it a news story about a space expedition or the political situation in a particular country, or was it a book review or interview with a film director? Why did your chosen article grab you? What questions did it make you ask? Why did you want to know more?

The serious student of economics, politics and the arts, should also check out their school or local library for: The Economist, The Statesman, The London Review of Books, The Times Literary Supplement, The Spectator. For online political commentary, Google The Huffington Post.

BOOST YOUR PERSONAL STATEMENT

ARCHITECTURE
- Visit inspiring buildings and make notes on why you find them interesting
- Keep up to date with new architectural methods and building techniques
- Study the work of one or two famous architects in great detail

Useful resources: 'The Architects' Journal', 'Architectural Review' and 'The RIBA Journal'

ART & DESIGN
- Visit art exhibitions and design shows frequently
- Choose a few favourite artists and designers both past and present and familiarise yourself with their body of work
- Get your family or friends to set you extra-curricular projects
- Learn how to use programmes such as InDesign and Photoshop

Useful resource: www.creativereview.co.uk
www.itsnicethat.com

BIOLOGICAL SCIENCES
- Read the New Scientist and National Geographic regularly
- Attend events such as the Cambridge Science Festival
- Research the work of at least three famous biological scientists

Useful resource: www.rsb.org.uk

BUSINESS / MANAGEMENT
- Read the Economist and the FT regularly; follow two or three stories in detail
- Participate in business challenges such as Young Enterprise, or the ICAEW BASE competition
- Apply for placements at small companies and get experience in a range of fields within a business (family or local is fine)

Useful resource: www.managementtoday.co.uk

CHEMISTRY
- Check the Royal Society of Chemistry website for updates on lectures and events you could attend
- Discuss how advances in chemistry affect our day-to-day life
- Read Chemical Week for the latest news

Useful resource:
www.chemistryworld.com

CLASSICS
- Read books such as The Iliad by Homer and The Aeneid by Virgil
- Learn basic Greek and Latin in your spare time
- Visit Hadrian's Wall or a similar historical site
- Listen to BBC Radio 4's programmes on Ancient Greece and Ancient Rome

Useful resource: classics.mit.edu

COMPUTER SCIENCE
- Set up your own website, even if it is just for fun
- Read Computational Fairy Tales by Jeremy Kubica
- Research a famous computer scientist such as Alan Turing and discuss their influence on the world today
- Look up and understand the four main concepts of computer science

Useful resources: www.livescience.com
www.cs.ox.ac.uk/geomlab

DENTISTRY
- Apply for work experience at a dental surgery
- Volunteer to teach younger children about dental hygiene
- Practice an activity that will demonstrate excellent manual dexterity such as painting, embroidery, playing a musical instrument or even having a go with electrical soldering kits!
- Read journals such as the Dental Update or Dentistry Mag

Useful resource: www.bda.org
www.healthcareers.nhs.uk

DRAMA & PERFORMING ARTS
- Try to get a prominent role in your school productions, whether on or off stage
- Visit the theatre as many times as you can, and compare the productions to film adaptations
- Read a different play every week and make notes on how you would direct key scenes
- Ensure you have knowledge of all genres, eras and styles of theatre
- Read reviews and understand how to critique them

Useful resources: www.thestage.co.uk   www.doollee.com

ECONOMICS
- Make notes on stories about the economy, both national and global, that interest you
- Research the potential economic consequences of Brexit
- Try to get work experience or attend an insight day at a leading financial firm
- Read the Financial Times and The Economist

Useful resource: www.res.org.uk

ENGINEERING
- Study five structures that you admire in great detail, and ensure you fully understand how and why they work
- Think about your favourite gadgets and what problem they solve
- Try and invent something that solves a problem, however small

Useful resources:
www.tomorrowsengineers.org.uk
www.raeng.org.uk
'Engineering Education'
or 'Applied Sciences,
Engineering Technology' publications

ENGLISH LITERATURE
- Read, read, read, read; not just novels, read plays and poetry too, of all eras and genres
- Watch theatre, television and film adaptations of the books you read
- Start your own book club at school

Useful resources:
www.literaryreview.co.uk
The Times Literary Supplement

GEOGRAPHY
- Research current global issues such as the environment and population – be able to discuss your findings in depth
- Become a member of the Royal Geographical Society

Useful resources:
'Geographical Association'
www.nationalgeographic.com www.rgs.org

HISTORY
- Visit historical sites, museums and exhibitions
- Read books, watch documentaries and even films set in historical times
- Demonstrate your understanding of biased and flawed evidence
- Carefully read the course syllabus: will you be studying ancient or modern, British or international, or a bit of everything?

Useful resources:
www.historytoday.com
www.royalhistsoc.org

HISTORY OF ART
- Read Critical Terms for Art History by Nelson and Shiff
- Listen to BBC Radio 4s' 'In Our Time' Culture Archive online
- Visit art galleries, make notes on the artists and their place in history

Useful resource:
www.metmuseum.org/toah

LAW
- Attend insight days run by law firms
- Volunteer to help out at your local solicitor's office
- Follow stories in the news of high-profile cases in a variety of areas (criminal, commercial, property, family etc.)

Useful resources:
'The Lawyer', 'Lawyer 2b' 'The Law Journal UK'
l2b.thelawyer.com

LINGUISTICS
- Ensure that you understand the difference between linguistics and languages
- Read Noam Chomsky's Syntactic Structures and Steven Pinker's The Language Instinct
- Practice some basic phonetics by writing down sentences in the phonetic alphabet

Useful resource:
www.sil.org

MATHEMATICS
- Research mathematical theory that is outside the A-Level curriculum, eg Fermat's Last Theorem, Euclid's Proof of the Infinitude of Primes, Pythagorean Triplets and Jordan Normal Form Theorem
- Enter the UKMT Maths Challenge and take part in MENSA tests
- Make notes on the ways in which mathematics can be applied in society such as engineering, economics and computer science

Useful resources:
www.lms.ac.uk
www.plus.maths.org.uk

MUSIC
- Read Marcus Du Sautoy's The Music of the Primes
- Research how music relates to mathematics, BBC Radio 4 has an archive programme on this
- Read Scales, Intervals, Keys, Triads, Rhythm, and Meter by John Clough

Useful resource:
www.musictheory.net

PHARMACY
- Get work experience at your local pharmacy or GPs' surgery
- Keep up to date on new drugs and advancements in the industry
- Read articles in journals such as The Pharmaceutical Journal and The British Journal of Clinical Pharmacy

Useful resource: www.learnhowtobecome.org/pharmacist

PHILOSOPHY
- Read Think by Simon Blackburn and The Problems of Philosophy by Bertrand Russell
- Watch TED talks online on the subject of philosophy
- Read up on the history of philosophy and the great philosophers

Useful resource: www.pfalondon.org

PHYSICS
- Regularly read the University of Oxford's science blog
- Keep up with developments from NASA and CERN
- Read and make notes on Lee Smolin's Three Roads to Quantum Gravity

Useful resources:
www.physics.org

POLITICS
- Read articles from Politics, Review and Talking Politics
- Show interest in local politics by volunteering at your local assembly and join your local Youth Parliament
- Set up a debating society at school
- Get a global perspective by reading international newspapers
- Keep up to date with global current affairs on a daily basis

Useful resources:
www.spectator.co.uk
www.theweek.co.uk

PSYCHOLOGY
- Read articles from the British Journal of Social Psychology and The Psychologist
- Join The British Psychological Societys' Student Members Group
- Attend lectures such as 'Psychology 4 Students' or attend a Psychology summer school at a leading university

Useful resource:
www.bps.org.uk

RELIGIOUS STUDIES
- Watch TED talks online on the subject of religion
- Ensure you can fluently discuss the beliefs and practices of all the main world religions
- Stay up to date on current affairs and how news stories have been affected by religious beliefs

Useful resources: www.ted.com/read/ted-studies/religion

SOCIOLOGY
- Read up on theories such as Marxism, Functionalism and Postmodernism
- Attend student lectures organised by the British Sociological Association
- Read articles from the British Journal of Sociology, as well as journals which relate directly to your interests

Useful resources:
www.sociologyonline.co.uk
www.britsoc.co.uk

VETERINARY MEDICINE
- Read Eckert: Animal Physiology by David Randall
- Attend events such as the London Vet Show or RCVS Question Time
- Volunteer for work experience with animals at your local vet or pet shop

Useful resources:
www.rcvs.org.uk
www.bva.co.uk

For any student taking any subject you must call your chosen universities and find out if they are running any summer schools, access programmes or open days for your subject. This will give a you the chance to really see what the course is like, and conveniently boosts your personal statement too. Sometimes, unis even reduce their entry requirements for students who meet a certain criteria and have attended outreach events. Contact your chosen unis to find out more!

University interviews

Will you have an interview? You need to do your research because some universities interview, others don't, and within individual universities, some faculties interview and others don't. Confusing!

We like to divide interviews into two distinct bits; the easy bits and the tough bits. The easy bits cover anything you can reasonably prepare for...

The easy bits

WHAT TO WEAR?

You want to feel comfortable but also look formal, but you don't want to be the only one wearing a three-piece suit! Most universities will inform you of the dress-code in the letter you receive with information about the interview, but adhering to the 'business casual' dress-code is a safe option. No denim, no trainers, no caps, no sportswear! You need to look like you're taking the interview seriously.

PLAN YOUR ROUTE AND ARRIVE EARLY

You'll be nervous enough so don't add any stress to your day. Plan your journey the night before so you know exactly where to go and how to get there. Remember to leave yourself plenty of time for travel. You are better off being early than late! Make a note of the department's telephone number in case of an emergency that causes you a delay.

READ UP

Go over your personal statement. The interviewer is likely to base questions on it as well as any academic work you may have submitted. You've effectively invited the interviewer to ask you questions on anything specific you mentioned, so you should revise any books, theories or other areas of interest thoroughly. Next thing is to look over the course syllabus for the university you are going to for interview (don't get the same course at different unis mixed up) and be as fluent as you can about the modules (both compulsory and optional) and how they are assessed.

SMILE

Sounds easy, but when we are nervous we lose our ability to control even the most simple facial expressions! Make sure you start the interview off with a nice big smile (not a demonic grin). Professors want bright students first and foremost, but they also want people that are friendly and will be a pleasure to teach.

SHAKE HANDS

A firm handshake goes a long way so practice this with friends at school – you want to come across as confident, not too weak or too forceful.

SMALL TALK

Your interviewer is likely to ask you some simple questions to break the ice, such as 'How was your journey here?'. Go into a little detail, it will help make you feel at ease and will hopefully build a rapport with your interviewer. Did you travel a long way? Say so! Did you get to see any of the campus on your journey in? If yes, tell them what you saw! Have you been to the university before, perhaps on an open day? Give us some detail! Don't be afraid of the old clichés about the weather either, that is absolutely fine and allows the conversation to flow, but whatever you do, don't give a one-word answer.

HAND MOVEMENTS

Playing with your hair, pushing your sleeves up and down and up again, fiddling with jewellery and biting your nails are all very common things people do when they're nervous. Worst of all they have no idea they are doing it… and it doesn't come across well. Practice what we call 'The Window'. Imagine a box the size of a laptop screen in front of your lap. Your hands must either stay on your lap, or occasionally go through the window and back again. This not only controls involuntary nervous twitches but actually helps you to convey passion and emphasise points.

BODY LANGUAGE

A great way to get comfortable is to practice sitting down. We know it sounds ridiculous, but bear with us. Sit on a chair in front of a mirror. Observe yourself. Where are your hands? How are your feet positioned? Are your legs crossed? Are you hunched over? Are your shoulders back, and is your chin up high? Are you sitting far back in the seat or right on the edge? What feels comfortable to you?

Do you look like a confident student looking forward to discussing your future studies, or do you look like a bag of nerves? Getting your seated position right before you go into the interview will help you to look and feel more self-assured when the big day comes.

Once you've established a comfortable position, start practicing some of the answers to the common questions – speak out loud. Having an answer prepared in your head is a great start but it's easy to get tongue tied…

QUESTIONS TO EXPECT

There are certain questions you can predict, and you should be ready for these. No-one should be surprised when they are asked why they want to study the subject, or why they think the course at that university is particularly good. Then there is the stuff you put down in your personal statement. The same goes for anything on the A-Level syllabus. It's not a test of knowledge – but you should brush up on any relevant current affairs, and have your own well-informed opinions.

"TELL ME ABOUT YOURSELF"

Remember, this is an academic interview, not a psychological evaluation. The interviewer is interested in information about you that relates to your degree choice. An obvious, but good place to start is your current educational situation, any hobbies that you have that relate particularly to the course, recent work experience and extra-curricular activities. Use your personal statement to help you to summarise yourself. You only need to give 4-5 sentences that you have practiced in advance.

"WHY DO YOU WANT TO COME TO THIS UNIVERSITY?"

Before you head to the interview you must do your research on the university, the town itself, the accommodation, the night life and societies and sports clubs that you can join. This will preferably have been done at the open day, but if for any reason you did not attend then you need to make up for it by showing the interviewer you know what you are letting yourself in for and have really thought about committing to three years or more at that particular institution.

"WHAT ARE YOUR STRENGTHS AND WEAKNESSES?"

It is highly likely this question comes up and it's one of the most important ones to be prepared in advance for, as you do not want to blurt out any undesirable traits in the interview! Really, the interviewer is looking for your strengths to relate to your course and that you do not have any fundamental weaknesses that would rule you out from studying it. For your strengths, think of skills such as communication, ability to adapt, determination, and organisation – and have an example of something you have done for each and every one of these. When answering the question on your weakness choose something that will not hurt you as a candidate, and explain what you are doing to work on it… for example, 'sometimes I am shy when meeting new people, but I have recently joined a local youth club which is quickly helping me to improve this'.

"ANY QUESTIONS?"

At the end of the interview, you may well be asked if you have any questions for the interviewer. Have some prepared. If you want to look like you are interested in the course and the university there really is no better person to quiz than your interviewer, and this will convey passion and enthusiasm. Here are some topics you could cover: how the course is taught, when examinations take place, number of lectures per week, how many students will be in the classes, is there support outside of lectures, what it is like living in the university city, the interviewers' background – did they attend the university? Make sure you don't ask any questions that should have been answered by the course prospectus as this will make you look like you have not done any research!

The tough bits

It's really important to make sure you master all of the easy bits, and practice those as much as you can, because the real challenge lies in the bit that is harder to practice – the difficult, unexpected questions designed to test your ability to think on your feet.

It really helps to understand what your interviewer is looking for, because the answer is often that they aren't just looking for the answer! Read on to find out what we mean.

LISTEN

It is amazing how many candidates do not listen to the question being put to them. It is also amazing how many students simply answer the question they would LIKE to have been asked. You will not be given credit for this and will give the impression of being a weak candidate with a few well-rehearsed answers. Once you've answered the question you can then steer the conversation onto topics you are most confident in, if relevant.

ASK

If there are any terms or words that you do not understand, do not try to guess, but ask for clarification. Often, if you are working through a complex problem, an interviewer will give you hints and tips to guide you towards a possible solution. If your interviewer makes a particularly forceful or intelligent point, incorporate it into your own argument or use it as a launch pad for further ideas. Try to make the experience as interactive as possible. Asking questions and asking for clarification on things you don't understand is a sign of confidence and shows a level of humility appreciated by admissions tutors.

BE HONEST

The interviewer might ask you a question for which you don't know the answer – don't panic! Ask them to repeat the question and if you still do not understand then be honest and explain to them that you don't know. If you make a point you later wish to correct or take back, let the interviewer know. Sometimes, there is no right or wrong answer and the interviewer just wants to gauge the way in

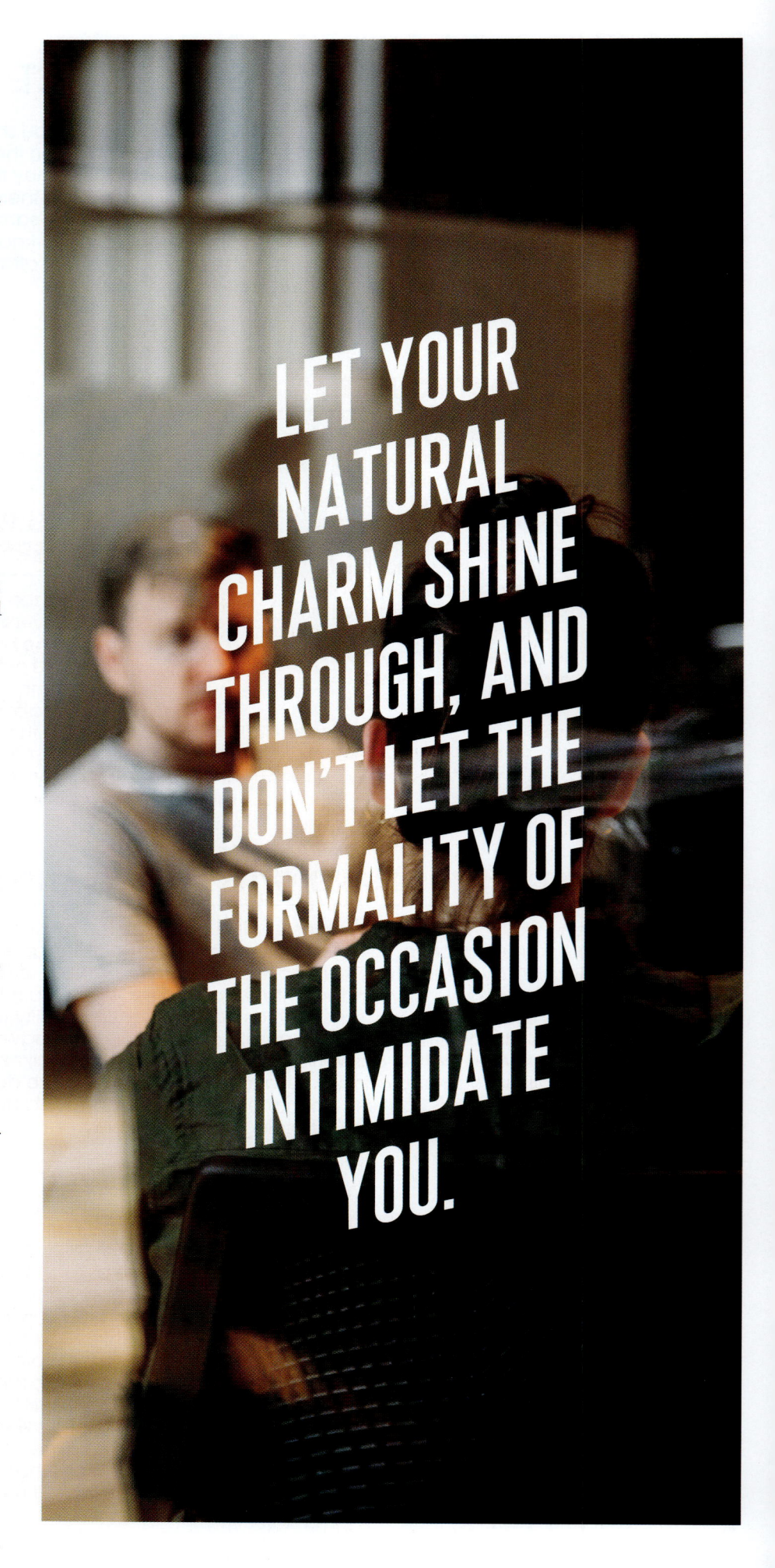

> LET YOUR NATURAL CHARM SHINE THROUGH, AND DON'T LET THE FORMALITY OF THE OCCASION INTIMIDATE YOU.

which you think, or the methods you use to come to an answer. You will be respected far more if you are honest about what you do and don't know. Also, a moment spent clarifying what is being asked of you will generally result in a better response to the question.

BE ENTHUSIASTIC

If you obviously relish the opportunity to discuss your area of interest with an expert in the field, it will be taken as a good sign of the genuine pleasure you take in your subject. So even if you get asked a question that truly stumps you, make it look like solving it is an enjoyable challenge!

BE CRITICAL

An ability to think logically and give concise, rational arguments will impress your interviewer so take a measured and intelligent approach to answering the question. How? Firstly, break it down into its component parts, if possible. Secondly, appreciate and acknowledge different sides of an argument. Thirdly, sit back and try to see why the question has been asked and where the interviewer is leading you. Don't be afraid to take your time and put your ideas in an ordered form before you begin to answer the question.

BE ORIGINAL

Throughout the course of your interview, you should be seeking not only to demonstrate what you know, but also to generate new ideas. Don't be too rehearsed, it's more about demonstrating potential than being polished. Use the questions as a stimulus to your imagination, and be bold in offering new solutions, suggestions or perspectives. As long as they are based on either facts or a logical argument, it does not matter whether your comments are ultimately 'right or wrong'. Feel confident in what you have to say, as you will never know everything (which is impossible!) but you can certainly use what you do know in a clever and original way.

What are they looking for?

MOTIVATION

How much do you really want to study your subject? Remember, your interviewer may have devoted his or her professional life to the subject you want to study for three years or more so they want to meet people whose passion reflects their own. Speaking with enthusiasm and discussing the variety of things you've done which are linked to your subject – both inside and outside the classroom – will make a good impression. Remember that nothing conveys passion as much as independent research and reading done in your own time.

POTENTIAL

Will you be better tomorrow than you are today? How about the day after that? And the day… you get the idea. Interviewers know that everyone has had different opportunities during their education, and they're going to try to look past your current level of ability into the future. The best way of showing this potential is by trying to respond intelligently to all the questions you're asked, especially the ones that you've never considered before or don't know the answer to straight away. Don't worry about gaps in your knowledge, just try to be logical and clear in your thinking.

TEACHABILITY

Are you going to benefit from the university course? Will you turn up to lectures and tutorials, and more importantly, will you learn anything whilst you're there? Will your lecturer find it interesting to teach you? Interviewers want to see someone with an inquisitive mind that's open and hungry for new ideas. Ask questions during the interview – it's a two-way process, and if you come out knowing something you didn't know before you went in, the chances are you will have proved your teachability.

PERSONALITY

Who are you? Are you going to be an asset to the university, and a fun and interesting person to spend three years or more with? Pretty obvious stuff: just let your natural charm shine through, and don't let the formality of the occasion intimidate you into clamming up. It may be of some comfort to know that very few interviewees manage to 'be themselves' in an interview situation, and nerves are the norm.

KNOWLEDGE

Most people think this is the most important thing you can possibly show at interview, but we find it's the least important of the criteria. The interview is NOT an exam. No one is going to just test you on what you know. Remember that the interviewer knows that everyone has experienced different standards of teaching: it wouldn't be fair or helpful to expect the same levels of knowledge from all candidates, or to use it as the sole measure of ability. However, remember that you must show the most important quality - motivation - through your love of the A-Level course, your outside reading, and further investigation of the subject. What would you make of someone who claimed to be a Liverpool fan, but had never heard of Steven Gerrard? If an interview meets someone with a total lack of knowledge, they are likely to interpret that as an absence of real passion for the subject.

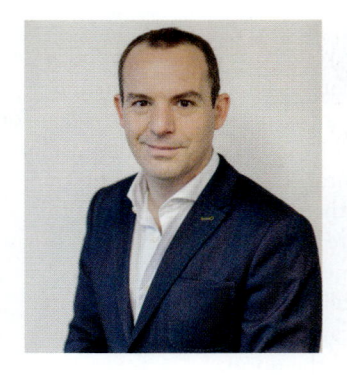

Student Finance

5 things EVERYONE should know
by Martin Lewis, MoneySavingExpert.com

Ignore everything you've read in the papers. Ignore the political spittle that flies across Parliament. And in some cases, ignore what parents tell you too. There are more myths and misunderstandings about student finance than any other subject (my polite way of saying there's a lot of bull spoken).

This is a political hot potato. People spin explanations to suit their own arguments. Yet that's about the big picture. When you come to decide whether you can afford to go to university, you should focus only on how it'll practically affect your pocket. And that is radically different to what you usually hear.

Now please don't confuse the fact I want to explain the system, with unblinkered support of it. I do have issues, but frankly that's not relevant here. What counts is that I tool you up to make the appropriate decision.

And another warning before I start. There was a radical change to student finance in England in 2012, anyone who started uni before that is on a different system, so beware their student finance war stories, that may not apply to you.

1. The student loan price tag is up to £50,000, but that's not what you pay.

Students don't pay universities or other higher education institutions directly. Tuition fees, typically up to £9,250 a year, are paid for you by the Student Loans Company. Over a typical three-year course the combined loan for tuition and maintenance can be over £50,000. But what counts is what you repay…

- You only start repaying in the April after you leave uni.
- Then you only need to repay if you earn £21,000+ a year (thankfully rising in 2018 to £25,000). Earn less and you don't pay anything back.
- You repay 9% of everything earned above that amount, so earn more and you repay more each month.
- The loan is wiped after 30 years – whether you've paid a penny or not.
- It's repaid via the payroll, just like tax and doesn't go on your credit file.

2. There is an official amount parents are meant to contribute, but it's hidden.

You are also eligible for a loan to help with living costs – known as the maintenance loan. Yet for most under 25s, even though you are old enough to vote, get married and fight for our country; your living loan is dependent on household (in other words, parents') residual income. The loan is reduced from a family income of just £25,000 upwards, until at around £60,000, where it's roughly halved.

This missing amount is the expected parental contribution. Yet parents aren't told about this gap, never mind told the amount. I wrote to the government asking them to change that – it refused.

So when you get your letter saying what living loan you get, you'll need to work it out the parental contribution yourself. Subtract your loan from the maximum loan available (eg for 2017 starters it's £7,100 if living at home, £8,400 away from home, and £11,002 away from home in London).

Of course some parents won't be able to afford it – and you can't force them to pay. But at least knowing there is a gap helps you understand what level of funds are needed. And it's important to have this conversation with your parents and discuss together how you are going to plug the hole.

In fact, while the papers often focus on tuition fees, I hear most complaints from students that even the maximum living loan isn't big enough. Funny isn't it, after everything that's said, the real practical problem with student loans isn't that they're too big, it's that they're not big enough.

So when deciding where to study, look at all the costs, transport, accommodation (and if you'll get into halls), as that's a key part of your decision.

3. The amount you borrow is mostly irrelevant – it works more like a tax.

This bit is really important to understand, as frankly it turns the way you think about student loans on its head. So take your time (read it a couple of times if necessary).

What you repay each month depends solely on what you earn, ie for now 9% of everything earnt above £21,000.

In other words the amount you owe and the interest is mostly irrelevant. As proof, for a graduate who earns £31,000…

- Owe £20,000 and you repay £900 a year
- Owe £50,000 and you repay £900 a year

- In fact, let's be ridiculous and say tuition fees have been upped to £1m a year, so you owe £3m+, you still ONLY repay £900 a year

So as you can see, what you owe DOESN'T impact what you repay each year. The only difference it makes is whether you'll clear the borrowing within the 30 years before it wipes.

It's predicted very few – only the top 20% highest-earning graduates – will clear it in time. So unless you're likely to be a seriously high earner, ignore the amount you 'owe'.

Instead in practice what happens is you effectively pay a 9% increased rate of tax for 30 years. At current rates, it works like this:

Earnings	Uni goers	Non-uni goers
Up to £11,500	No tax	No tax
From £11,500 - £21,000	20%	20%
From £21,000 - £45,000	29%	20%
From £45,000 - £150,000	49%	40%
£150,000	54%	45%

This doesn't make it cheap, but it does mean that all the talk of burdening students with debt is misleading. The burden is paying 9% extra tax – frankly it shouldn't be called a debt, it really doesn't work like one.

The more you earn, the more you repay each month. So, financially at least, this is a 'no win, no fee' education.

4. Interest is added, the headline rate is 6.1%, but many won't pay it.

Student loan interest is set based on the (RPI) rate of inflation – the measure of how quickly prices of all things are rising and it changes annually each September, as follows…

While studying: RPI + 3%, so this year 6.1%
From the April after leaving: It depends on earnings. For those earning under £21,000 it's RPI, for those earning over £41,000 it's RPI + 3%. For those who earn in between it's a sliding scale.

So many graduates aren't actually charged the full 6.1% rate. In fact many graduates won't actually pay any interest at all.

That's because the interest only has an impact if you'd clear your initial borrowing in full over the 30 years before it's wiped. Many won't. And even of those who will, all but the highest earners won't come close to repaying all of the interest added.

5. The system can and has changed.

Student loan terms should be locked into law, so only an Act of Parliament can negatively change them once you've started uni – but, they're not. And a few years ago we saw a very bad changed imposed, though thankfully after much campaigning it was overturned.

So sadly all my explanations above need the caveat of 'unless things change'.

This is just the start, if you'd like to read my full 21 student finance mythbusters go to www.moneysavingexpert.com/students/student-loans-tuition-fees-changes

> **USEFUL RESOURCES**
>
> UK: www.gov.uk/student-finance
> Scotland: www.saas.gov.uk
> Wales: www.studentfinancewales.co.uk
> Northern Ireland: www.studentfinanceni.co.uk
> Channel Islands: www.gov.je and www.education.gg
> The Isle of Man: www.gov.im

Budgeting

by Jake Butler, Student Money Expert at Savethestudent.org

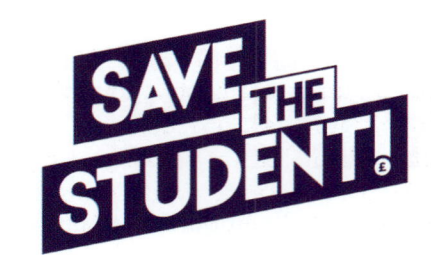

I've been part of Save the Student ever since I graduated, so I've always been knee-deep in student money and what it takes to survive at uni. What I've found from speaking to 1,000s of students is that budgeting is the secret. It's at the centre of everything you do that involves money at uni and day-to-day life! If you've already experienced budgeting before heading to uni then that's great, if not you're about to. Every new student must face one sooner or later. It sounds boring but it doesn't have to be, so before you turn the page make sure you give my budgeting advice a go. You won't regret it.

Why your cash is like a leaky bucket

A bank account is a bit like a bucket of water: every now and again you turn the tap on and fill it up – and then you've got lots of water! Unfortunately, your bucket has a few holes in it so, over time, you'll notice the water draining out of the bottom. The aim of the game is to always ensure you've got enough water so your bucket never runs completely dry – you want to plug the gaps, or get more water.

That's budgeting in a nutshell – and it doesn't get much simpler than that! Your bucket is your bank account (or your wallet, or wherever you keep your cash). The holes are whatever you spend your money on, and the tap is your income stream. Budgeting is the art of managing the leaks so you've always got enough cash to get by. No one wants a dry bucket!

Build a better budget

While there's lots of advice out there about what to do with your cash, the best budget for you is the one does what you need it to do. Without wanting to get too Zen on you, the art of budgeting comes from within – so your money plan will depend on what kind of student you are or want to be.

Some students budget from the top down: they separate their Student Loan (or wages) into neat weekly chunks as soon as it graces their bank account. For many others, budgeting is more of an accidental – usually after blowing a whole Loan instalment in one truly amazing weekend, and then having a tenner a week to live on for the rest of term.

Here's the bottom line: whichever side you come down on, you'll still need to budget – it has a way of catching up with you. Taking charge of your money (before it takes charge of you ...) is a much better place to be!

Budgets aren't Set in stone

How much you need, want or have to live on is different for everybody. It depends on things like:

» How much Student Loan, wages or other income you get

» Personal spending habits

» Hobbies

» The town or city you live in

» How often or how far you have to travel to uni (or home for the holidays)

» How much you spend on your social life

Watch out for those nasty bumps in the road too, including Christmas, birthdays, summer festivals or being butter-fingered with expensive gadgets (think dropping your phone for the 5th time). Any budgeting pro will set aside an emergency fund for these kinds of things.

Not all bumps are nasty, though! You might have more money coming in at certain times: getting birthday cash, work bonuses, or when your Student Loan lands in your account.

What that means is the best budgets are flexible. A bit like that bucket of water, some holes can be plugged or patched over, you might sprout new leaks – and you might find bigger tap to top it up!

Life is all about variety and the unknown: there's no reason why that has to stop when you get to university!

Getting into the nuts and bolts

It's time to get the pen and paper out, or word on your laptop if you prefer.

1. Write down and tot up all your income streams – Student Loan or uni funding, top-ups from your parents, wages from part-time job and anything else you can think of.

2. Then go ham and write down every single thing you spend money on.

It also helps to split these into two broad types: your fixed costs (such as rent, bills & food and variable costs (which need to be estimated) such as groceries and socialising.

Meanwhile, your main income streams can probably be counted on one hand: student loan, parent hand outs, part-time job…

In the case of the student loan, it's usually paid in 3 instalments throughout the year. The best thing you can do is to split it into the separate months throughout the year otherwise you'll have £1000s coming in on certain months of your budget sheet andbut sweet zero (and a 'dry bucket') on others!

Use a budget template

Here's a very quick and easy budgeting template to get you started. Once you get more confident you can start using Excel on your computer to level up your budget (and to add over the top colours to it).

EXPENSES	AMOUNT PER MONTH (avg)
Rent	(£395)
Electricity / Gas	(£50)
Water	(£8)
Internet & home phone	(£20)
Mobile phone	(£24)
Insurance (contents, phone, etc)	(£12)
Food & essentials	(£125)
Books & stationery	(£30)
Travel	(£44)
Clothes	(£24)
Socialising	(£70)
Anything else	
TOTAL SPENDING:	

INCOME:	AMOUNT PER MONTH
Student maintenance loan	(£600)
Parents' allowance	
Part-time job	
Savings interest	
Anything else	
TOTAL INCOME:	

	AMOUNT PER MONTH
Total income	
minus Total spending	
Equals a MONTHLY BUDGET OF:	

Freshers' Week

For some, Freshers' Week is an exhilarating seven days sparkling with new faces and fizzing with the taste of freedom. For others, it can feature people and experiences you spend the remaining three years trying to avoid. Your first week at university is an exciting, bizarre time; there is a lot that can – and should – be crammed in. Here are a few tips to live it out to its full potential.

People

Ok, so you don't know anyone. Everyone else seems to have made loads of friends already and you worry you will never make any. You see yourself eating alone in the canteen every day and they'll all point and laugh… The first thing you need to know about Freshers' Week is that no one really knows anyone very well and no one knows what to expect or who to talk to. But everyone is keen to look like they do. Try to talk to as many people as you can, even if you hate small talk. Go with the flow and try to keep an open mind. University is a melting pot and there is every chance that you'll befriend people very different to those you would have expected to before you arrived. Don't expect meaningful relationships to blossom immediately but enjoy the panoply of personalities and their quirks.

Events

Your social calendar will be awash with parties, fairs and events. Go to as many as possible, they are an excellent way to meet people. You may have to put up with cheesy student anthems and wear some oversized t-shirts but it'll be fun.

Registration

You will queue for hours to have a mug shot taken for your student card. Use your student card liberally. It gains you entry to all student nights, and discounts on tickets, clothes and music – among other things. When in doubt, flash it.

Lectures & Tutorials

Yes, you'll have to go to some of these in the first week. They are important in terms of getting your bearings, establishing what you'll be studying and catching a glimpse of your fellow classmates. Some more progressive tutors like to play 'ice breaker' games, so if you dread the thought of being caught on the spot, you best know what to say about yourself when it's your turn in the introduction circle. If you're nervous about your academic ability compared to others, don't be. You are there because the university wants you there.

The Freshers' Fair

All universities have clubs and societies that use the fair to sell themselves to you. They offer a mind-boggling array of extra-curricular activities for you to follow up on old hobbies, beliefs, activities, or to branch out and try something new. There is no time after university in which you will have such eclectic opportunities – make the most of them. They, too, are a great way to make friends. Sign up for anything that seems interesting - you can always change your mind later.

Halls

Halls are noisy. People like to crank up their stereos, sing, play games and shout about their crazy antics. In Freshers' Week, the fire alarm might go off every five minutes; burnt toast and drunken fools the likely culprits. It's annoying, but if the alarm sounds, make sure you still leave the building. And, it's not unusual for traffic cones and street signs to appear in the common room. (This is illegal though, so try to bring home some legitimate mementos instead).

Love

You will probably not find it in the first week (although there are always couples who meet on day one and are together three years later, and beyond!). Enjoy it, with all its bumps and potholes. It's all part of the experience.

Your Room

Hall rooms can be a bit spartan. The Freshers' Fair will probably have on offer innumerable posters and potted plants to spice up your domain (remember to water the plant). And the bed linen provided will look less than inviting so, if you can, bring your own.

Washing

The same rules apply as at home. You have to wash (yourself and your clothes). There'll be a laundrette nearby, and some halls will have washing machines so there is no excuse!

Hygiene & Health

Take care with what you eat, try to have a balanced diet and remember basic health and safety precautions in the kitchen are as essential at university as in the wider world, if not more. Make sure to look after yourself — especially during the first couple of weeks if you want to avoid getting struck down by 'Freshers' Flu'. To stay feeling your best, try to get plenty of sleep and fit in some exercise. Oh, and try to get ahead of others by registering with the doctors during Freshers' Week; there is usually one on campus.

Feeling Lonely

Everyone will experience this in the first few weeks of term at least once. It's perfectly normal, but if you feel like it's getting too much then speak to Student Services - if you have trouble coping with anything at university, there are many resources to help you, no matter what the problem. Find out what they are and where they are.

And finally – your family misses you. Call them from time to time.

Making the most of your time at uni

It's tempting to laze your free afternoons, weekends and summer holidays away, but beware – the job market is competitive and you're going to have to do something to show that you're worth employing when graduation comes around. Here are some tips to help you maximise your spare time at university and set you apart from other graduates when you are looking for your first full time job.

Institute of Student Employers — ise.

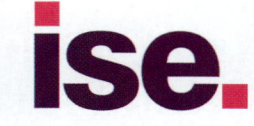

With thanks to Stephen Isherwood, CEO of Institute of Student Employers

During term time

Whilst at university there are services set up to support you to develop a career plan and gain new skills. Usually they are free (which they may not be once you graduate) so make the most of them while you can.

VISIT THE CAREERS GUIDANCE TEAM
Use all the resources available and don't leave it until your final year - you will be much too busy doing your final exams to think seriously about it then. A significant number of employers now offer spring weeks to first years, open days and internship programmes that can all be accessed before your final year.

SET YOURSELF REGULAR CAREERS-RELATED OBJECTIVES
For example, exploring potential career opportunities, understanding your strengths, finding relevant work experience, developing a draft CV and gaining practical interview skills.

LEARN TO SELL YOURSELF
Marketing your own skills often doesn't come naturally but is a critical skill that you need to develop. Use every opportunity to build these skills, for example, join your debating society or do a presentation skills course. Use the language that employers speak. You don't have to approve of business jargon but you do need to know what employers are talking about when the time comes to start job hunting.

DEVELOP YOUR SKILLS
Employers want to see real skills that you can apply in their business. These may be people skills such as leadership or self-reliance skills such as networking. Sign up for as many skills workshops as possible. Look out for any careers related modules or options.

EMBRACE THE OPPORTUNITY TO JOIN CLUBS AND SOCIETIES
Take part in new activities, sports, clubs and societies. It will give you a chance to meet new people, build your self-confidence and develop key skills. In today's competitive world you need much more than just qualifications.

During summer holidays

Use your summers wisely. They are the longest holidays you'll ever get. Most students have up to four months off – this is plenty of time to get some work experience or an internship, and have time to work to save the pennies for the year ahead, travelling or your future plans.

WORK EXPERIENCE AND INTERNSHIPS
Work experience will show employers that you are proactive, diligent and, above all, serious about a career. Try to seek out paid internship opportunities, or a structured volunteering programme. You will develop skills by meeting new people and being in a working environment. You will be able to add career-relevant, bright, sparkling experience to your CV whilst learning more about your career options.

TRAVEL
Students often use their long holidays to travel. If you are interested in seeing more of the world, and experiencing different cultures and environments then grab your passport and venture off the beaten track. This world of ours has a million and one things for you to see and do beyond our shores. Travelling can be expensive, but you could fund it through part time work, or by working for half of your holiday and saving your pennies. You could also look into volunteering opportunities abroad; save turtles in the Galapagos, help build a village in Africa or teach English in Indonesia – this is rewarding, useful and impressive.

Employers want to hire people who are motivated, passionate about what they do and have the intellect and skills to get things done. By focussing on your studies and your extra-curricular activities in a meaningful way you will get the career opportunities you seek.

Changing your course or dropping out

Changing your course

You applied to do the course, spent hours agonising over getting your personal statement just right, celebrated when you got an offer and have finally arrived at your university, excited to begin the first of three or more years studying a course you thought would inspire you and take your knowledge and understanding of the subject to dizzying heights.

But you don't think you like it, it's not what you thought it would be and you just can't get inspired. You're not alone - each year 16% of students across the UK decide to change their course or university.

If you are not enjoying your chosen university subject because it is too difficult, assessed in the wrong way for you or not what you had expected, you might be considering changing course. Some students find that once they start university, they change their mind about their future career path, and require a different subject.

Make sure that you speak to a careers advisor or tutor at your university to get their advice on the options available to you. They might have a way of solving your problems without having to go through the difficulties of changing your course.

If you decide to change course, you will usually have to restart your degree from year one, and so you will be at university for longer and will rack up more debt in tuition fees. It will also be longer before you get a job. Some courses will have specific grade requirements for entry into their department, so you will need to check this before you contact the relevant professors.

Dropping out

Students drop out of university for various reasons. It is a very serious decision to take, particularly in terms of the financial implications, and therefore one that you should consider carefully. Just like changing a course, it is very important to contact your careers advisor and tutor to ask their advice. Are there any courses that you would prefer doing instead of this one? If your decision to drop out is due to health or personal reasons, would you consider returning to university after a year? After discussion with your tutor, it is usually possible to take some time out to reconsider your options.

If you have made the decision to drop out of university, there are two main options available to you:

– Reapply to a different university to start the following year. This would be a good idea if you like the idea of university, but were not enjoying life at your particular institution.

– Get a job or apprenticeship. There are many exciting career opportunities available for school leavers. Read through the alternatives to university section.

Things to consider

Enquire
Speak to Student Services and find out what your options are – they will have heard this all before so don't feel that they will judge you or that you are inconveniencing them. Whether you want to change course, university or even take a year out, they will be able to help you with all aspects, including student finance as your loan or grant may be affected.

Research
You will need to do your due diligence and research the new course you have in mind thoroughly. Go and find the faculty, speak to staff as well as current students of your new chosen subject and get a very clear idea of what it entails. Be prepared to defend your decision because you may be asked to explain why you have chosen your new subject.

Make a list
It is a good idea to draw up a list of all the things that you like about your course, and the things you dislike. Then write a list of all the things you like about the university in general, and the things you dislike. Compare them and see where there is overlap – this will enable you to see if it is the course or the university that you want to change.

100% sure?
If university life is not what you expected, changing the course may not help. It's very important that it is the course itself you are not enjoying. Be careful not to confuse homesickness, loneliness, stress, or poor time management with wanting to change your course. If these issues are what's on your mind then speak to Student Services who will be able to help you.

Don't delay!
After you have made a definite decision you need to get the changes made quickly so that you can start your new course as soon as possible – the longer you leave it the more catching up you'll have to do.

Working for your uni

"My name is Michael Keohane, I am a third year Journalism and Creative Writing student at the University of Roehampton. I also work with the University as the Digby Stuart College President representing thousands of students in Roehampton's biggest college.

I moved to London a young 18-year old country bumpkin who had just left his hometown of Baltimore, West Cork in Ireland. Going from a village of 500 people to a university of over 9,000 was really daunting but I had a gut feeling it was going to be worth it.

Roehampton welcomed me with open arms, making sure that I had lots to do and lots of friends. There was something to do almost everyday and I really quickly forgot all form of homesickness. Instead I was just excited for each new day.

My classes were nothing like school, which for me was so important. I didn't hate school but it also wasn't my favourite place in the world. University showed me that learning can be fun and practical which I loved and spurred me to get more involved in Roehampton life.

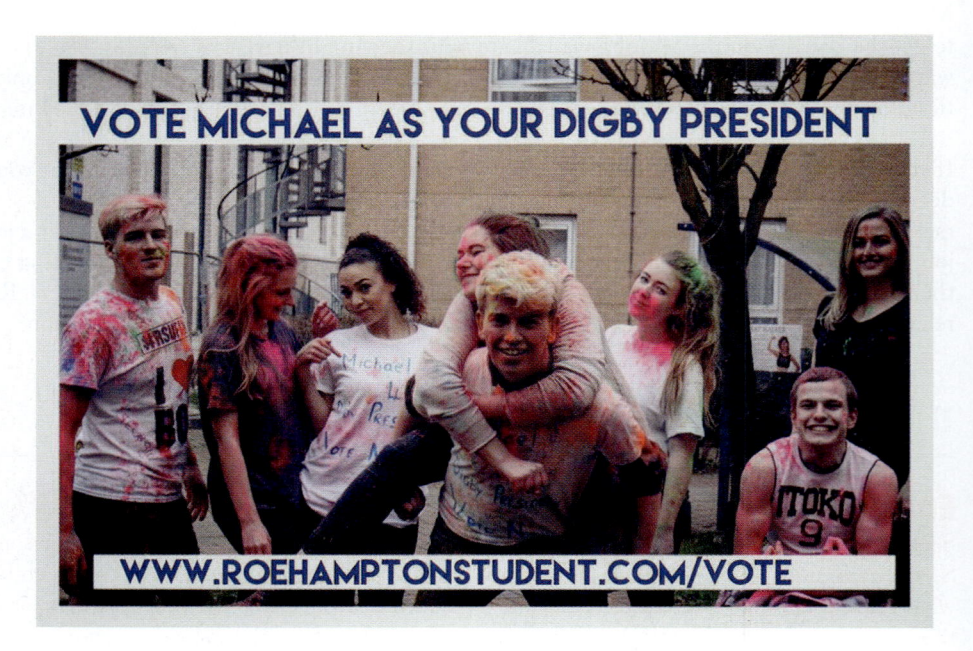

When I first started university I was rather shy, it was a huge opportunity for me and I was terrified that I may mess it up.

After a week or so however, I quickly realised it was about to become the best experience of my life.

Michael Keohane

Student – *Roehampton University*

I quickly began volunteering for RAG (Raise and Give charity work) and the media team at the Student Union. By second year I had a weekly television show for the SU and was the vice-chairperson of the Student Activities committee.

The university also made sure that I wasn't short of money by giving me a job as a student ambassador which was helpful in so many ways to make sure I could treat myself but also pay for basic necessities.

As my second year drew to a close I decided to run in the Student Union elections and run to be the president of the college I was apart of. This was a two-week long experience of canvasing, putting up posters, making videos and spreading the word to students on why I would be best for the role. The election had a HUGE turnout and I found out that I had won my category so was elected the President of Digby! This meant that I represented all the students in Digby for any issues that arise for them and fight to make sure that they are well treated throughout their time at Roehampton.

My role has led me to meet loads of people, some of whom are helping me hugely in seeking employment after university. I sit on meetings with the directors of the university and get to make changes that will effect future generations of Roehampton students.

The role doesn't come without it's perks either! Being the president means I get free rent in on-campus accommodation and also get to go to some events for free to meet lots of lovely new people!

I think if I were to give one piece of advice to a university student it would be that what you put into university is what you get out of it. My time at Roehampton has been incredibly busy but rewarding in so many ways and prepared me for the working world so that I am confident to go straight into my field.

I wouldn't change my university experience for the world - I hope that you won't either!"

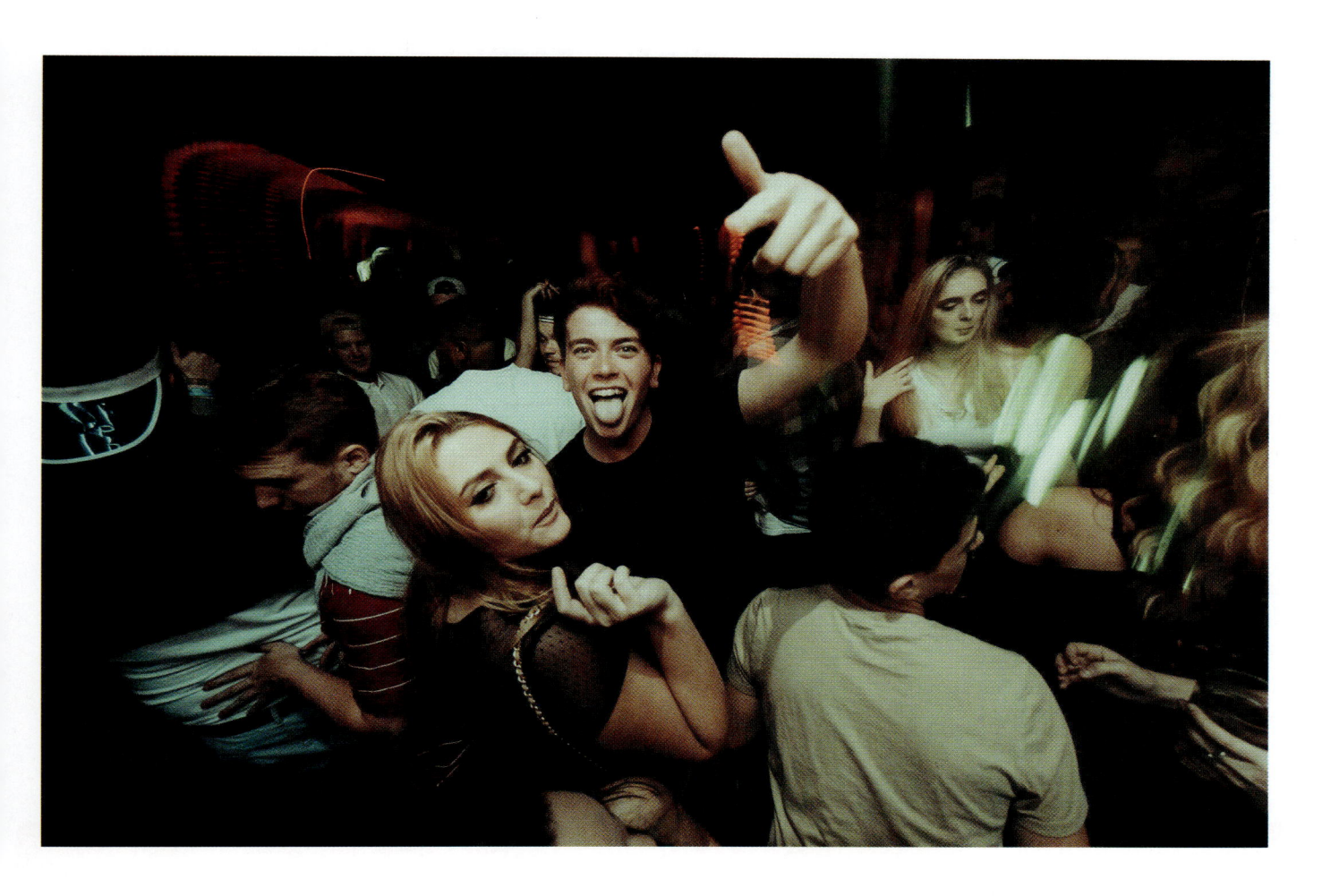

A GUIDE TO DEBATING

What is debating?
Debating is just arguing with rules, where both sides have an equal opportunity to speak and convince the audience. The essence of debating is trying to persuade people of your point of view, setting out a coherent set of arguments for why you should or shouldn't do something. There is also a chairperson, who acts as a mediator, to make sure that it is fair and everyone has the opportunity to speak.

Examples of debates
There are formal debates such as in the House of Parliament, Question Time, Presidential debates in the US elections, and in School Council. Likewise, there are less formal debates such as on such as talk shows and panel shows.

Not just a shouting match
The key difference between a debate and just a shouting match is that only one person ever speaks at any one time, so everyone has a chance to speak. This is also the one distinction that you need to have in debate sessions at all times. You give them a chance to speak, and then you will have a chance to speak.

Not like a boring lecture or speech
Unlike a lecture you get an opportunity to respond and engage with what the previous speakers have said. You get to question them and show why what they said is wrong. Of course you cannot argue against them unless you listen to what they say first; it is therefore critical to engage with the other side's arguments during the debate. This is what makes debating exciting.

About Debate Mate
Now in its tenth year, Debate Mate is a global educational organisation that teaches key skills of communication, critical thinking, and eadership through debating. Each week 6,000 students participate in Debate Mate across the UK, USA, and Caribbean, and over the past nine years, more than 30,000 young people have benefited from our programme.

Visit our website: www.debatemate.com

DEBATE MATE

WHAT ARE THE RULES?

Every debate has a motion - a statement. One side, the proposition, argues for the statement. The other side, the opposition, argues against it.

Each side has 4 speakers, who take it in turns to speak. The 1st proposition speaker speaks first, followed by the 1st opposition speaker, the 2nd proposition speaker, and so on. These speeches are 3-5 minutes long.

After the 3rd opposition speaker has spoken, there is a floor debate. Members of the audience may make short speeches (up to 2 minutes each) to which the teams in the debate may not respond to at the time.

Following the floor debate there are summary speeches given by the 4th speaker from the opposition, and then the 4th speaker from the proposition. NB: The summary speeches are reversed – the opposition speaks first, and the proposition has the last word. These speeches are 3 minutes long.

The diagram below shows the order of a debate:

PROPOSITION ↔ **OPPOSITION**

FLOOR SPEECHES

WHY DEBATE?

Debating develops your ability to convince people of your view or make them agree with you, and speak in public.

Debating is about effective teamwork - which means you learn to work with different people who have different opinions, which can help to develop your own. This is a really important skill which you will use throughout your life in school, college, university and work.

In the future, you will find that schools, colleges and employers are looking for people with the ability and confidence to communicate their ideas, think quickly on their feet, question and assess ideas, work in teams and who have an understanding of the issues that affect our lives. This is exactly what debating equips you with.

Most importantly debating is a lot of fun, you get to discuss important issues that you care about in an exciting and engaging way!

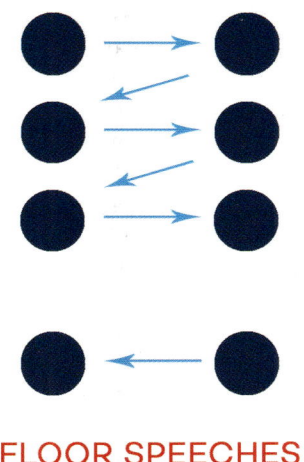

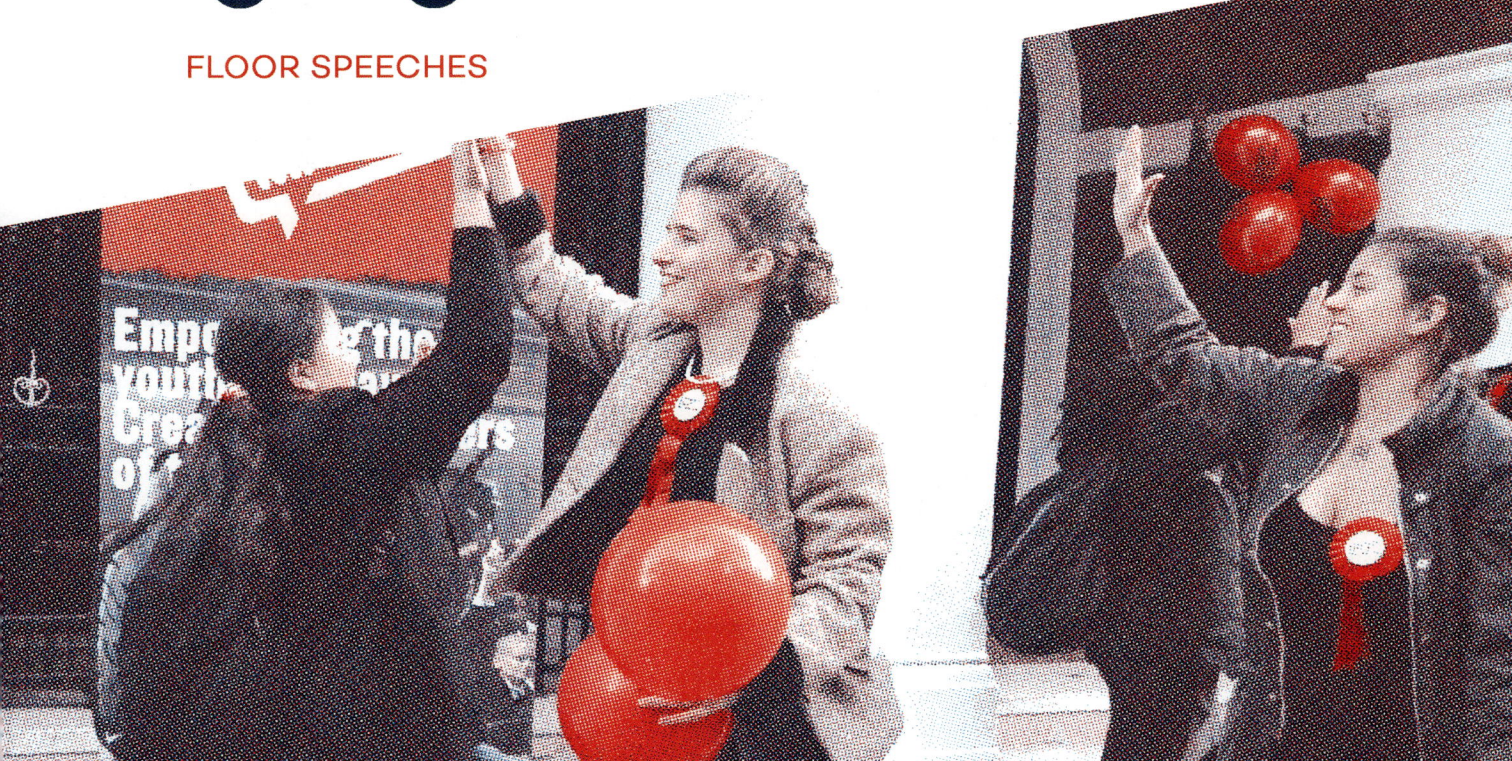

Studying abroad

Packing your belongings, saying farewell to friends and family and immersing yourself in a new culture, environment and even language to study your degree is a brave move indeed, but one that will be recognised and rewarded in years to come.

By taking on such a challenge you will be demonstrating that you are adaptable, culturally aware and resilient. You will also be opening yourself up to unique, exciting international opportunities, perhaps learning a new language, making friends from all over the world and expanding your employment opportunities upon graduation infinitely.

If you are interested in studying abroad there are lots of different options, you don't have to go away for the full duration of your undergraduate degree. It might be that you would prefer to be based in the UK but travel abroad for just one year of your degree. We've explained some of the options below to help you decide which might suit you best.

Full degree (3-4 years)

Studying at a university abroad for the full duration of your degree will bring huge benefits. You'll live in the city you study in, immerse yourself in the culture, speak the language and make life-long friendships over the course of three years. The first step of the challenge is to find out which course you want to study and where. Most other countries don't have a central system like UCAS to make it easier for you, so you will have to apply to the universities individually. If you are applying to study a course that will be in another language you will have to show proficiency in that language, so just like with UCAS personal statements, make sure your applications have no mistakes. There are many organisations out there to help you.

Term/semester (5 months)

You can choose to study abroad for one semester of your degree, this will be around 5-6 months. This will still give you an enriched experience, but your main degree will be awarded by a UK based university. Your classes for that semester are conducted abroad and you live in the city you've chosen for the entire semester. This option is great for students who want to test the waters of studying abroad.

Summer school (1-2 months)

Lots of universities offer summer schools for anything between 3-8 weeks. There is often a charge to these summer schools, but they will give you a chance to use your summer wisely by studying in a different country and meeting people from all over the world. These aren't tied into your undergraduate degree and you can study any subject that you are interested in.

Sandwich courses (1 year)

If you like the idea of studying abroad, but going away for your entire degree seems a bit much then you should consider sandwich courses, where you spend only part of your degree course in another country.

Depending on the course you choose at university, some students will also have the opportunity to take a year out as part of their degree – this is particularly true for language students, joint honours degrees and many business courses. You can take time out independently or as part of a scheme.

Erasmus (1 year)

The Erasmus Programme is an EU exchange student programme that has been in existence since the late 1980s. Its purpose is to provide foreign exchange options for students from within the European Union and it involves many of the best universities and seats of learning on the continent.

The programme is aimed at cross-border cooperation between states to aid the growth of international studying, and with over 4000 students involved in the programme at any one time it offers an excellent chance of experience abroad.

Students must be registered in a higher education institution and enrolled in studies leading to a recognised degree or other recognised tertiary level qualification (up to and including the level of doctorate). There is no immediate change to the UK's participation in the Erasmus+ programme following the EU referendum result and the UK National Agency will continue to manage and deliver the programme across the UK.

All participants and beneficiaries should continue with their Erasmus+ funded activities and preparation for the published application deadlines until further notice.

How will I fund it?

Once you've decided you'd like to study abroad, the next hurdle that you need to overcome is funding. Student loans are not available from the Student Loans Company for students who wish to study outside of the UK. Students from the EU pay the same fees regardless of which EU country they are from, however individual countries do not have to give financial help unless the student in question has been living in the country for at least five years. If you wish to study outside of the EU, tuition fees are generally much higher and will need to be paid upfront.

So, how should you tackle the funding issue? Firstly, check the tuition fees at the university you wish to attend, and then approach the appropriate agency in the country you wish to study. Make sure that you know exactly how you are going to fund your studies before you apply, and take the time to research bursaries and scholarships that may be available to you. You'll also have to think about how you fund your accommodation, food, social life, and all the other expenses that students incur. You should definitely consider getting a part-time job whilst you study, or working during the holidays in between terms. You could also take out a personal loan from your UK bank, but it is important to bear in mind that you will have to repay the loan immediately and that your bank will charge you interest.

If you are planning on studying outside of the EU, you must check whether you will be permitted to work whilst studying as this is not always the case. Please ensure you look into funding as soon as possible, if you have even a small inkling that international study could be for you, then start researching straight away to find out what is possible.

How will Brexit affect me?

Fees for British students will be the same as those paid by other EU students until the UK officially leaves. There is less certainty about what will happen after Brexit, especially if Britain leaves the European Economic Area (EEA).

But it's important to consider different EU countries separately: a change to fees is unlikely in Germany, for example, since study there is free to students of all nationalities. In other EU countries, though, individual governments or institutions may take a harsher stance on British students' fees.

THINGS TO CONSIDER

VISA – Will you need a visa to study in your chosen country and how much does it cost?

LANGUAGE – Will the course be taught in English, or will you need to demonstrate proficiency in another language?

ACCOMMODATION – Will the university help you find accommodation or will you have to organise this yourself?

LEAGUE TABLES – Have you looked at the international university rankings?

COSTS – What are the average costs of living in your chosen country?

VISITING HOME – If you are studying on the other side of the world, it might not be easy to travel home during the holidays, so consider how often you might want to come home and include the cost of flights home in your budget.

USEFUL RESOURCES

STUDY IN THE US:
www.fulbright.co.uk

BURSARIES & SCHOLARSHIPS:
ukcisa.org.uk

STUDY IN AUSTRALIA & NZ:
www.studyoptions.com
www.studyingdownunder.co.uk

STUDY IN EUROPE:
www.thecompleteuniversityguide.co.uk/international/europe
www.erasmusprogramme.com
www.european-funding-guide.eu
www.eunicas.co.uk

FOR ALL OTHER COUNTRIES:
idp.com

Studying in the USA

Have you ever considered studying in the US? You're not alone: more than 11,500 students chose to study in the US last year. There are many options to fit your interests and finances, from a full bachelor's degree to a summer internship or study abroad programme.

Read on for more information about these options and ways the US-UK Fulbright Commission can help you achieve a place at an American university.

Why go abroad?

Why do so many students cross the Atlantic? In a recent survey, we found British students were most attracted to the availability of funding for undergraduate study in the US, as well as the reputation and flexibility of its degrees - you don't have to choose a field of study until your second year. Studying or working abroad for a summer or semester is also a fun and exciting way to learn about a new culture, all the while expanding your CV and developing the international perspective and skills employers seek.

Your options: A bachelor's degree

You may have heard US study is expensive or that it is difficult to apply. First, keep in mind that Fulbright's advising team has many free resources and events on American university admissions. Also, millions of dollars in scholarships and financial aid are offered each year on the basis of your academic success, financial need or for being an international student. Over 250 alumni of the Sutton Trust US Programme have access to $68 million in funding.

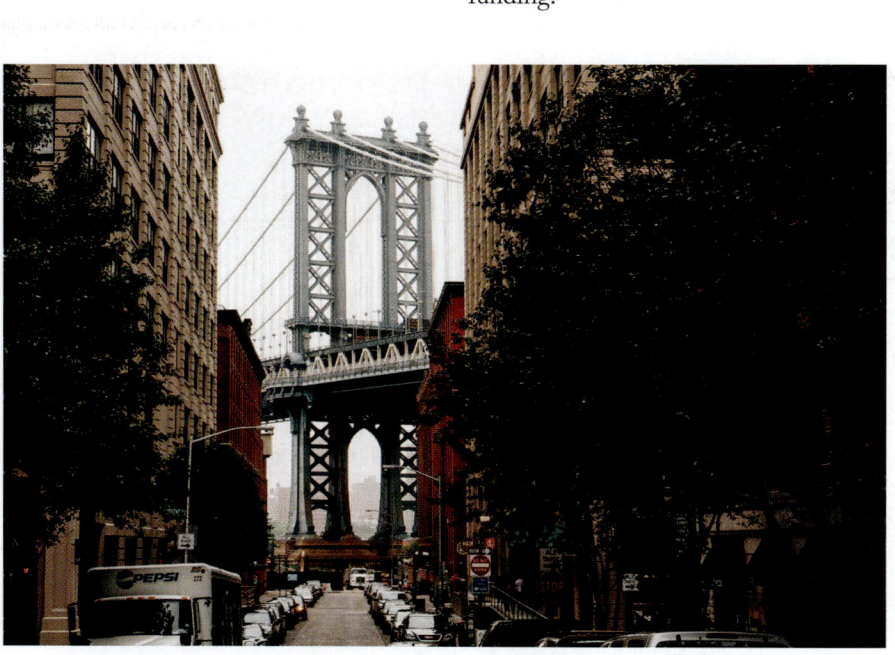

Study abroad and internships

If you complete your degree in the UK, there are still plenty of opportunities to go to the US. Most UK universities have programmes set up for you to spend a semester or year abroad at an American university. You'll be able to use your UK loans, and your tuition fees are discounted for the time you are abroad.

If you're interested in a summer programme, Fulbright offers two Study of the US Institutes, hosted by American universities for UK undergraduates. Another option is to explore short-term work opportunities during your UK degree, such as a summer camp or internship programme.

What are you waiting for?

Check out the Fulbright website – www.fulbright.org.uk – for step-by-step guides on US undergraduate admissions, internship programmes and Summer Institutes. If you are planning to study in the US for a full degree, come along to our USA College Day Fair on 28-29th September 2018 and meet reps from over 180 US universities, or attend a Fulbright seminar on undergraduate study.

The Fulbright Commission also partner with the Sutton Trust US Programme (us.suttontrust.com), which helps British state school students apply to American universities through support, advice and a one-week summer school in the USA. It is free to take part in the programme.

Studying in Australia and New Zealand

Australia and New Zealand share much with the UK – a language, a history, and an education model. While universities there are a long way away, being a student down under is much the same as it is here.

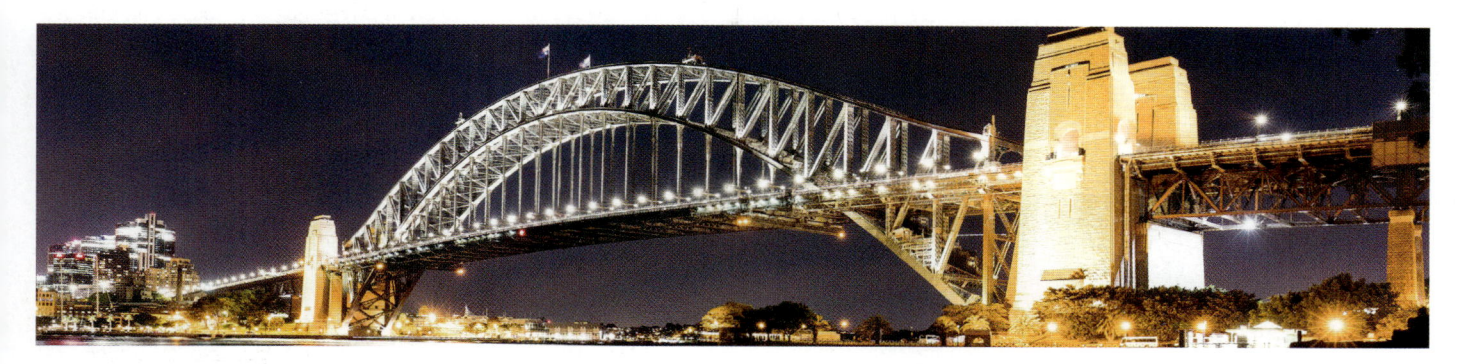

Their degrees are directly equivalent to a UK degree. They take the same time to complete and are taught in the same ways. Australian and New Zealand universities have all the facilities you'd expect at a good UK campus, including libraries, cafes, laboratories, bookshops, bars, Student Unions, sports facilities and student clubs and societies.

For all these reassuring similarities, however, there are key differences. It is usually these that attract UK students.

Broad, flexible degrees

Undergraduate degrees in Australia and New Zealand are broader than UK degrees. When you enrol on a general degree (a Bachelor of Arts, Bachelor of Science or Bachelor of Business) you will choose a 'major'. This is your specialist subject. You can also study subjects from outside your major ('electives'). This allows you to construct a degree that is unique to your interests and tailored to your goals.

Teaching culture

Contact teaching hours in New Zealand and Australia are higher than at universities in the UK and the teaching atmosphere is relaxed and informal. UK students in Australia and New Zealand report that academics are accessible and easily approachable if they have questions or problems.

Student life

The universities offer a huge range of opportunities for you to make the most of your student years. You can go on academic exchange, do an internship, join a community project, get involved with a student society, or take part in a leadership programme. Or all the above!

Prestigious, world-ranked universities

Many students are drawn to studying in Australia and New Zealand because of the reputation of their universities. In the 2014-2015 QS World University Rankings, 9 Australian and New Zealand universities are ranked in the world's top 100, compared to 19 from the UK. There are only 42 universities in Australia and 8 in New Zealand, compared to around 120 in the UK.

Australian and New Zealand universities are seen as world leaders in a diverse range of subjects including sport science, physiotherapy, geology, physical geography, social work, environmental science, and marine studies. They also offer amazing opportunities for fieldwork. Marine scientists in Australia, for example, can use the Great Barrier Reef as a living laboratory…

THE PRACTICALITIES

COSTS AND FUNDING
You will need to budget for tuition fees and living expenses for the duration of your course.

Each university sets its own tuition fees for each course so universities charge different amounts for the same degree. Check tuition fees carefully. The least expensive courses are lecture-based (for example, history or English literature). The most expensive are medicine and dentistry. Fees start at around £9,000 per year.

For more information on Australian and New Zealand universities, see: www.studyoptions.com/scholarships-and-funding.

HOW AND WHEN TO APPLY
Applications to Australian and New Zealand universities should be made through Study Options, not via UCAS. Applications to overseas universities should not be listed on the UCAS form, and do not impact your chances of getting a university place in the UK.

You can apply to up to five universities in Australia and New Zealand via Study Options. These are in addition to your UCAS choices.

Studying in Europe

Despite being closer geographically, and certainly much cheaper to get to, than the US, New Zealand, or Australia, the main consideration when studying in Europe will be language. If you aren't already proficient in the local language of your chosen destination, you may view this as an exciting challenge to acquire an excellent new skill, or it may raise concerns about settling in. Some unis offer what is called 'English Medium Tuition' courses which means you will learn your degree in English, alternatively you can throw yourself in the deep end and learn alongside local students in the local language.

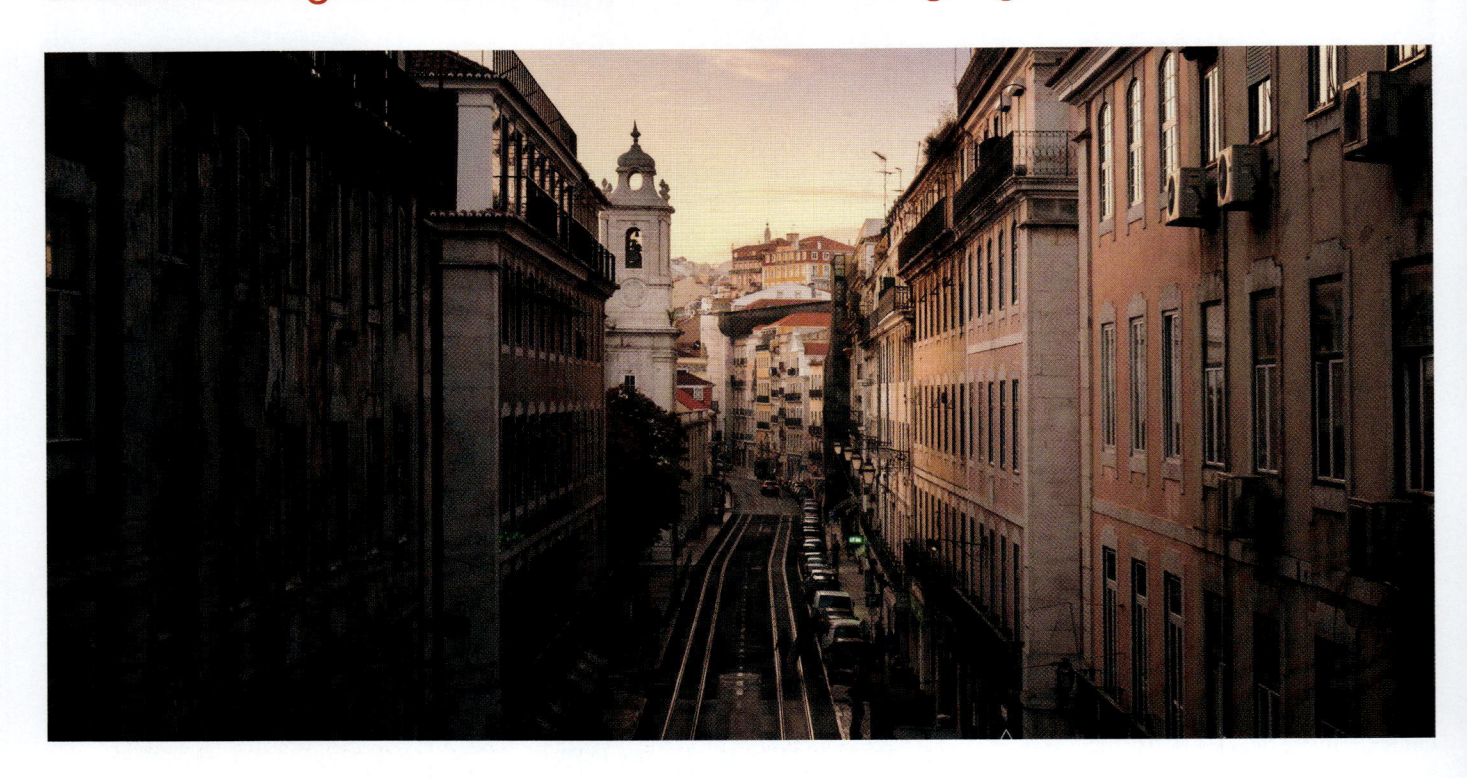

Culture

You will be hard pressed to find a place more rich in culture than Europe! Art, music, literature, architecture, ancient history and modern politics can all be explored with relative ease and low cost. Many students spend their holidays interrailing - adventures by train across the continent. What better place to study history then in the very places it happened?!

Funding & entry requirements

The good news is that many countries in the EU charge much less for their degree programmes than on home turf.
The even better news is that the entry requirements for many courses are lower than UK universities. This isn't necessarily a reflection of quality - the UK university system is disproportionately oversubscribed, but make sure you don't choose a course just because the grade requirements are low! You'll need to research the institutions individually, and see how they do on league tables, as well as get some insight into the university experience from UK alumni - the uni should be able to put you in touch.

Which country?

If you already have an affiliation with a European country, perhaps family roots, an interest in their history or culture, or you have already begun learning the language, then that may help to sway your decision. If you are just keen on exploring Europe and don't have a preference, then let the course and quality of the institution be your guide. Although you will no doubt have many wonderful experiences and meet life long friends wherever you go, when the course is finished you will want a quality degree from an internationally recognised institution to show for it.

My Experience

STEF SILVESTER
studies in New Zealand

"I am studying a Bachelor of Science, majoring in biochemistry, at the University of Otago in New Zealand. I decided to study in New Zealand because of their similar education system and because I'd always dreamed of travelling here!

Dunedin has a student population of 25,000 and there is always something to do with so many students about. There is a great range of clubs and activities from tramping and kayaking to dancing and knitting. Nightlife is a huge part of student life here. Most weekends a good party can be found by following the music!

My classes are great. I can access all my lectures online as well as via podcasts. The labs are really well-equipped and there is plenty of help available if needed, through study groups or one-on-one tutor sessions.

Coming to New Zealand is one of the best decisions I ever made and I'd urge anyone to make the same jump!"

OLIVER BROOM
lived in France for a year during his degree

"I chose to spend the third year of my Durham University French degree course in Grenoble, France. It seemed the perfect opportunity for me to experience living abroad at the same time as trying to become a fluent French speaker.

I organised it through my university. I had to fill out some forms requesting to go to university in Grenoble and Student Services gave me guidance on the whole process. I spent the summer before working hard and saving to supplement my student loan. In September I moved into an apartment which was found for me by my host university, Université Stendhal.

I had an amazing time and met people from all over the world, English speaking, French speaking, and many others, and I am still in touch with many. Studying French at a university in England is all very well, but it is no substitute for immersing yourself in another culture, language and way of life day in day out.

So it was fantastic socially and did wonders for my French, but I have also since found out that employers look very favourably on graduates who have spent time living abroad, and since graduating I have found it comes up again and again in interviews. I would definitely recommend the experience to anyone."

IBRAHIM BUTT
Duke University
(Class of 2020)

"Two years ago I started an incredible journey with the Sutton Trust US Programme that culminated in my acceptance to Duke University in Durham, North Carolina. Studying abroad was always going to be a priority during my undergraduate degree and the programme inspired me to contemplate completing my whole degree in the USA. I was given expert advice and support on all aspects of the challenging USA university application, and have never regretted my decision to study in the USA!

The main attraction of the USA was the liberal arts system of education on offer, which is completely different to the UK system. I've been able to take classes ranging from foreign languages to theology, allowing me to discover my interests before committing to a degree path. When submitting my applications, I had no idea which degree subject I wanted to do, so the US system and its flexibility has allowed me to engage in different subject areas before choosing my degree!

My experience in the US has been unbelievable, from hiking in the Appalachian Mountains as part of an orientation programme, to being served breakfast at midnight before our final exams by my professors - the sense of community on campus is inspiring. I am surrounded by diverse individuals from over 70 countries who are involved in all parts of campus life.

There's much more than just academics at an American university, especially so at Duke. Students are encouraged to change their campus, community and country. Opportunities include fully funded summer trips around the world to engage in community service projects, from environmental conservation to volunteering in schools.

My time in the USA has been phenomenal; the academic freedom and school spirit offered at US universities are unrivalled and I cannot wait for what the next three and a half years have to offer!"

HARVARD UNIVERSITY

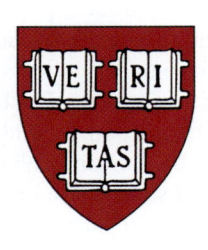

You have probably heard of Harvard College, located in the USA in Cambridge, Massachusetts, but do you know how to prepare for and apply to an American university?

Harvard has created a website especially for British students, teachers, and parents/guardians – all the information you need to educate yourself about US unis, about how to apply, what kinds of students go there, and especially about Harvard.

Just go to www.harvard-ukadmissions.co.uk and find out for yourself what the opportunities are!

And don't be put off by the US uni fees – make sure you read the "Financial Aid" page and see how the generous Harvard scholarships programme can often provide enough support so that the costs are actually competitive with the UK. Below are some of the typical questions Harvard often hears from British students – we answer them more fully on the website, where some current and former students give their views and comments too.

What does a "Liberal Arts" programme mean?

Liberal arts is an American term for an academic programme that recognizes the need for both broad education across the spectrum of the arts and sciences and depth of education in one specific field. You do not apply to a specific programme, but instead just "apply to Harvard" and then choose your particular field of interest, or "concentration" during the second year of the four year programme.

What are some benefits of the American college experience?

Student diversity: You can expect to find classmates from all across North America and around the world, coming from every conceivable socio-economic, geographic, religious, ethnic, and political background. The diversity of experience and belief and the resulting exchange of ideas add to the lively mix of campus life, both in the classroom and outside. After graduation, you'll have friends and contacts all over the globe.

Extra-curriculars: Most colleges in the US encourage a balance between your academic and extra-curricular lives. Schoolwork is primary, but your outside interests are equally important. Make friends, practice organizational skills, learn the fine arts of team-work, diplomacy, and compromise – all while having fun!

Residential life: Harvard, like many US colleges, provides on-campus housing for all students for all four years, which means that 24/7 you are surrounded by the social and academic life of the school.

Timeline: Start your search for information early!

There is a degree of forward planning involved in order to assemble all the required information in time for the deadlines, so it is helpful to think about this process as early as Year 11 or even before. The application deadline is January 1st for entry the following September. You will also need to take some standardised tests called the SATS (no relation to the UK ones!) or ACT, and because they are in multiple-choice format, it is a good idea to practice them in advance. Have a look at the website that discuss the application process and the application requirements such as the SAT or ACT tests.

Getting the Application together

Grades: There are no set grade cut-offs for admission, but for the most selective colleges in the US, such as Harvard, usually GCSE's would be mostly A or A*, and predicted A-Levels would be AAB or better. This past year we had over 37,000 applications for about 2,000 places...you do the maths! But also remember that Harvard is not just about grades, but seeks out exceptional all-rounders.

Essays: You will need to write personal essays as part of the application. The website offers you some good examples of US-style writing.

Recommendations: Two teachers plus your housemaster or careers advisor should write letters of recommendation on your behalf. Ask them to include as many details and anecdotes as possible to help bring you alive to the reader. There are samples of good "Teacher Reports" on the website too!

Interview: You will have the chance to meet informally with a graduate of Harvard. The dual purpose is to let you ask questions of someone familiar with our campus and community, and for us to learn more about you. We talk more about this on the website.

Uni Costs and Harvard's Financial Assistance

It's true that Harvard is more expensive than Uni in the UK, but in many cases financial assistance will be sufficient to make the "net price" affordable. Harvard is fortunate to be able to admit all students, even international students, without regard to whether they need financial assistance. We have a generous financial assistance programme which awards bursaries based entirely on need and not merit, and takes into account all costs (tuition, fees, room, board, books, and travel.) We want to be sure that the best students, no matter what their economic background, are able to enrol at Harvard. More details about our financial assistance programme, including typical aid awards for UK families and a link to our easy-to-use Net Price Calculator can be found on our website:

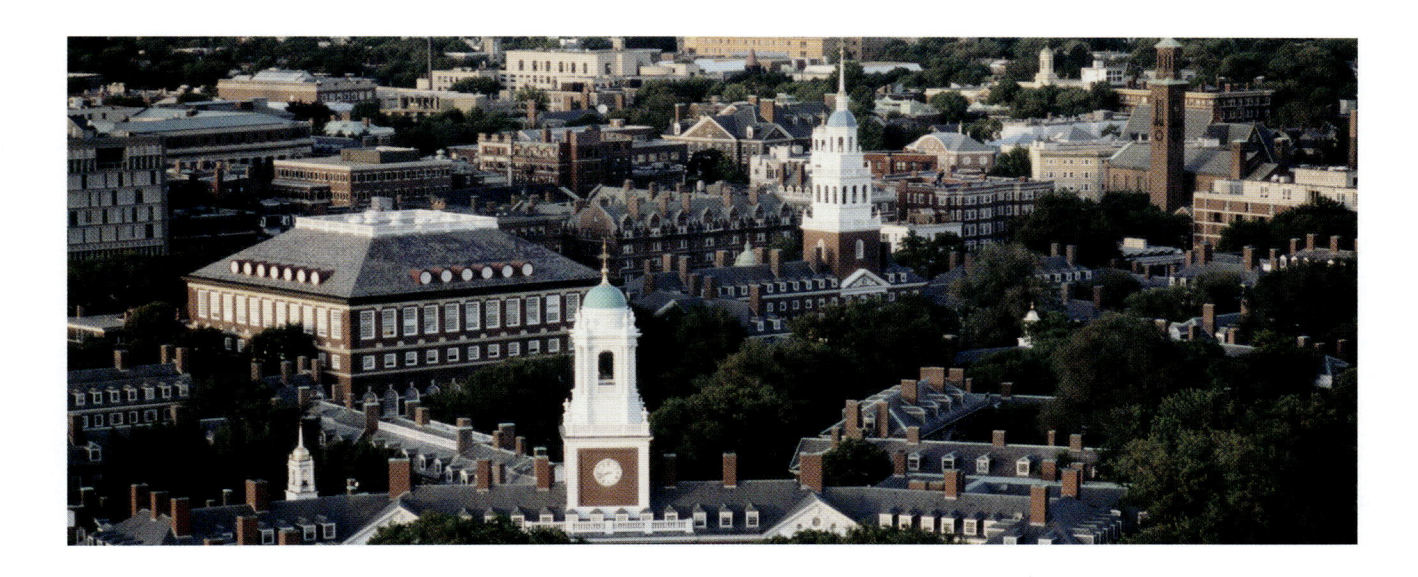

Net Price Calculator: college.harvard.edu/financial-aid/net-price-calculator
Admissions: college.harvard.edu/admissions
Financial aid: college.harvard.edu/financial-aid

www.harvard.edu

Gap years

We are asked again and again what universities and employers think of students taking gap years. The majority of universities and employers we work with really don't mind either way and some actually prefer for students to take gap years as it helps students to develop a wealth of life skills. That said, it's worth noting that in some rare case academic departments within universities that would advise against taking a gap year, so have a conversation with your potential universities before you launch into planning your year out.

In most cases, students consciously plan to take a gap year, but for some it might be unanticipated. Here are some of the top reasons why students take a year out:

1. Travel

Whether you are interested in seeing the pyramids, want to work on a conservation project in South America or you plan on exploring the Great Barrier Reef, a gap year is the perfect chance to satisfy the travel bug within. The time between school and university provides a really great opportunity to go and do these things before you're committed to longer term education or careers.

2. Results

You might be forced to take a gap year because your A-Level results weren't quite as good as you had expected, and you now need to retake some of your exams and reapply to university. Don't worry – this is not uncommon and your school or college will be able to offer support.

3. Work

If you're career-minded, a gap year can be a great way to gain a valuable placement to add to your CV. There are plenty of employers offering gap year work placements but you need to start researching these in year 12, as most employers will expect you to apply during year 13. You should receive a salary, which is great as it means you start university with some extra cash in your bank account or have some money to spend on travel, a car, or anything else you might need.

4. Time to reflect

You have been in full-time education since the age of 5, which can take its toll. Some students need to take time out to think about what it is they want to do next, be it university, a school leaver programme or entering full-time employment. A gap year can offer you the time you need to think about your options, rather than jumping too fast into something which isn't right for you.

Whatever your reasons for taking a gap year bear in mind that universities and employers will expect students to be productive with their time, so don't just think that you can spend a year glued to your parents' sofa. Speaking of parents, we suggest you have a chat with your family before you plan your gap year – although it is your choice, it's worth asking for their advice and keeping them in the loop. They might have already planned on turning your bedroom into an office, gym or walk-in wardrobe, so you might want to let them know that you will be sticking around for an extra year!

Some students we speak to are concerned about taking a gap year and being left behind when the rest of their friends head off to university. But its worth considering that this is your chance to do something for yourself; to take a year out to do things that interest you; that helps you develop your skills and gives you life stories that you will want to share with your grandchildren!

USEFUL RESOURCES   volunteerics.org   etrust.org.uk/the-year-in-industry   realgap.co.uk   vsointernational.org   projects-abroad.co.uk

My Experience

STEPHEN SPENT HIS GAP YEAR GAINING EXPERIENCE IN INDUSTRY:

"After my original gap year plans to go travelling didn't come to fruition I knew I still wanted to do something exciting and worthwhile with my year out. Having already deferred my place at the University of Southampton to study engineering, I wanted to do something related to that field. I wrote to and called a number of companies but all were a bit reluctant to take someone on with limited professional experience and qualifications.

For any STEM subject, one of the best ways to find a worthwhile year of experience is through the 'Year in Industry' scheme. I filled out a single application form, which was then sent off to all kinds of big-name employers in the engineering sector including: Rolls-Royce, Aero Engine Controls, BAE Systems etc. A few weeks later, there was an interview day in which all these kinds of companies were present and they invite you to attend a 15 minute interview. If they're interested in you then they'll contact you for a further interview at their own offices and from there they'll send out offers.

I was offered a placement with Rolls-Royce, working on their gas turbine engines. The scheme is designed to ensure you get the most out of your placement and you are therefore given target-focused projects which make a real contribution to the department you are in. A lot of my work focused on improving manufacturing processes and saving costs, this meant I was often presenting to high-level management and suppliers. Although this can be very daunting at first, it was undoubtedly the most worthwhile experience I have had for developing my personal and professional skills.

I was worried that the year out may affect my ability to go back to university the year after and study again. However, I believe the year in industry gave me a better focus and an insight into the area I want to go into in the future. In my summer holidays I've been able to go back and work at Rolls-Royce, proving my placement to be useful for making contacts in the industry and securing further work to contribute towards my CV. Overall I would thoroughly recommend a year in industry before going to university as it has given me a massive head start compared to my course mates, whose first taste of industry will be in their first real job."

JO SPENT HER GAP YEAR TEACHING ENGLISH IN A SECONDARY SCHOOL IN TANZANIA:

"In between my first and second year of A-Levels I was able to travel with my school to volunteer in Costa Rica for one month. During that trip I realised how much I enjoyed travelling; seeing new places, meeting new people and learning about different cultures and traditions and as soon as I got back I knew I wanted to see more of the world before going to university so I decided to take a gap year. I still went through all the usual university application process in Year 13, going to university open days, writing my personal statement and applying through UCAS but I chose to defer my entry by one year on my application form. At the same time as applying to university I also had to decide where to go and what to do during my gap year - at that point, the world really was my oyster! I knew I wanted to go somewhere different from home, where I could volunteer and feel part of a community so I chose to volunteer as an English teacher in Tanzania, East Africa. As soon as I finished my A-Levels I worked full time for 5 months to save up all the money I needed to go away. Before my placement I was matched up with another volunteer and we travelled out together to a secondary school in the foothills of Mount Kilimanjaro which would become our home for the next 8 months. The teaching was very rewarding and being able to learn about the education system in a different country was really eye opening. Although it was a huge challenge, I learnt so much from a different way of life - we had no running water in our house, electricity but only for a couple of hours a night, we had to hand wash all of our clothes, cook on a small paraffin stove and had a 1 hour walk to get to the weekly food market! During the school holidays we travelled around Tanzania and other parts of East Africa and I even got to take a group of 15 students to the top of Mount Kilimanjaro as a geography field trip! The experience changed my outlook on life and education forever, and I would urge anyone who is thinking about volunteering abroad to get out there and do it, you won't regret it!"

LEARN ABOUT CAREERS DIRECTLY FROM INDUSTRY LEADERS!

GENERATE London hosts free after-school talks for teens in central London. Meet innovators from tech, business, fashion, media, law, medicine and more. Hear their exciting personal journeys and take part in candid Q&A sessions.

PAST SPEAKERS

Dr Henrietta Bowden-Jones: *Psychiatrist and Addiction Specialist*
Matthew Ryder QC: *Barrister and Deputy Mayor*
Jake Davis (aka Topiary): *Former Hacker*
Amber Atherton: *Entrepreneur*
Dynamo: *Magician*
Sean Langan: *War Correspondent and Filmmaker*
Tiffanie Darke: *Magazine Editor*
Tom Hollander: *Actor*
Thomas Heatherwick CBE & Stuart Wood: *Designers*
Sir Harpal Kumar: *CEO Cancer Research UK*
James Gay-Rees: *Film Producer*
Bejay Mulenga: *Social Entrepreneur*
Ella Woodward: *Food Writer Deliciously Ella*
Oli Barrett MBE: *Entrepreneur*
Parker Liautaud: *Arctic Explorer and Environmentalist*
Anya Hindmarch CBE: *Fashion Designer*
Richard Reed CBE: *Co-founder Innocent Drinks*
Alex Klein: *Co-founder KANO Computers*

GENERATE
LONDON

GENERATING IDEAS   CONNECTING TEENS   INSPIRING CONVERSATIONS

generatelondon.co.uk

APPLY

CAREER
PROFILES

APPLY

2018

"What are you going to do with your life?"

This is a question you have no doubt been asked a thousand times by teachers, parents, family friends, and relatives who think you should have mapped out your future by now and be able to summarise it in a sentence. In reality, not many people know what they're going to want to do in two years, let alone ten years down the line – but it is something to start thinking about. Now a decade into our careers, the Pure Potential Team have some advice to pass on...

When our grandparents embarked on their careers times were very different. The old-fashioned, traditional roles of husband going out to work while housewife looks after the house and children is only one of a plethora of lifestyle options that we can choose today. And when these husbands of yesteryear chose their career path they would usually stick to it, often staying within the same company throughout their entire working life, gradually rising up the ranks until retirement. Oh, how times have changed.

So, next time someone asks you 'what are you going to do with your life?', translate the question to 'what's your next step?'. These days it is much more common for people to try out several different careers throughout their lifetime, taking sideways steps into different industries and retraining to gain new skills. When choosing which career path to take it is so much more daunting if you feel like you are being forced to decide the rest of your life. So, instead think of it one step at a time, each step giving you more experiences to find out what it is you really enjoy. And believe me you will find it eventually, if you don't get complacent and stay in a job that doesn't inspire you.

I have friends who are over 30 who still aren't sure, but they try different roles and with each new experience they are fine-tuning what it is they really want to do, and they are enjoying the journey of discovery. Take my friend Sophie for example – she went to university, did her law conversion course, got a training contract with a top law firm, worked there successfully for several years ... until her 29th birthday when she decided after all that that her real passion lay in film. She did some work experience, met as many people working in the industry as she could, then quit her job and is now working for an independent film production company and loving it. Best of all she is able to use her legal knowledge to look after the legal side of the business, such as drawing up contracts with actors and film crew.

Sophie's story is a great example of how the skills you learn in one job can be transferred to the next. So don't worry that embarking on a career will mean that you are stuck in it for life. The most important thing is that you pick up skills such as working well with people and getting along with clients and colleagues (communication skills), getting on with your work without your boss having to keep asking you (self-motivation), working out what can be improved - from the filing systems to the sales strategy to the day-to-day efficiency of the rest of your team – and acting on it (taking initiative), being willing to work late sometimes or cover for a sick colleague or take on new responsibilities (flexibility), that you won't forget what you need to do, or lose important documents (organisational skills) and that you know how to use a computer (IT skills). Any job from doctor to fireman to marketing manager to PR officer to lawyer to banker to entrepreneur will need every single one of these skills.

Don't forget also that your life outside of work will change with the years, and so too will your needs. In your twenties you might want to work in a fast-paced environment, with the opportunity to travel, meet new people and live in the city surrounded by bars, restaurants and nightlife. If you get married and have children you may decide that you want a quieter life, and that travelling isn't going to be practical. Everyone is different so don't do what your peers do, or what your parents expect. There is a job out there for you that you will love. Maybe not every minute, but something that you fundamentally enjoy and gives you a sense of achievement and fulfilment, whatever that may mean to you.

So, during which moments do you feel most fulfilled? Is it when you score a goal in football? What about when you hand in your big coursework project? Or when you are out with friends and making them laugh? Is it offering advice to someone in the year below you? Or helping a friend during a difficult time? Reading a brilliant novel? Performing or speaking in assembly? Think about those moments and then think laterally, not literally. If you enjoy scoring a goal in football it doesn't necessarily mean you should become a professional footballer, but it could mean that you enjoy working in a team, thinking on your feet and getting results in high-pressure environments, so you could be suited to a role in sales. If you really relished the moment you handed in your coursework after months of working on it then perhaps you are more suited to a more research-based role, such as investment management, or law. If you enjoy being the centre of attention amongst friends then maybe you'd be suited to a job where you have to charm clients – something like equity sales at an investment bank, or as a management consultant gaining the confidence of CEOs. Do you see where we are going with this? Think about what you enjoy and then apply it to job roles, in a 'big picture' way... and this can literally be anything. If at this time in your life the only time you feel happy is when you are at home on your sofa watching boxsets on Netflix (you'd be amazed at how many students we meet who say stuff like this) then you are likely to be suited to a role based in an office, which doesn't have to be boring!

When you wake up every day, and go to work from 9-6 or beyond, you need to be sure that your job is giving you a sense of personal fulfilment and satisfaction. We don't mean that every day you spring out of bed, desperate to get back to your desk and sing good morning to your boss, but we do mean that when you get asked if you enjoy your job you can reply 'YES' with conviction. Take our jobs at Pure Potential for example, helping state-educated students to pursue their dream careers and get into the world's best universities makes us happy. This feeling of achievement doesn't have to be charitable though, it could be that you get a real buzz from problem solving, creativity, adventure, justice or the advancement of science and technology. Only you know what is important to you, so have a think about what you believe in and what your values are.

What we will say is that the better the grades you get now will stand you in good stead for future job security and a higher salary. So work hard, even if you're not sure what you're working for and keep your options open.

As your life twists and turns through the remainder of school, possibly a gap year, a university degree, a school leave programme or apprenticeship, keep an eye out for careers that might suit you. Everything in life, from taking transport to school, the food you eat, the magazines and books you read, the television programmes you enjoy, the money you spend, the shops you spend them in, the home and community you live in, the countries you visit, has hundreds, no, thousands of jobs supporting them... one of which will be right for you.

> We don't expect that after reading this article you will now have a definite idea of what you want to do next, but we hope that you will start to have a sense of yourself and your skills and a clearer understanding of what sort of things you should be thinking about when deciding on the next stages in your life.

USEFUL RESOURCES

www.themuse.com
www.learnhowtobecome.org
www.prospects.ac.uk

FREE ENTRY

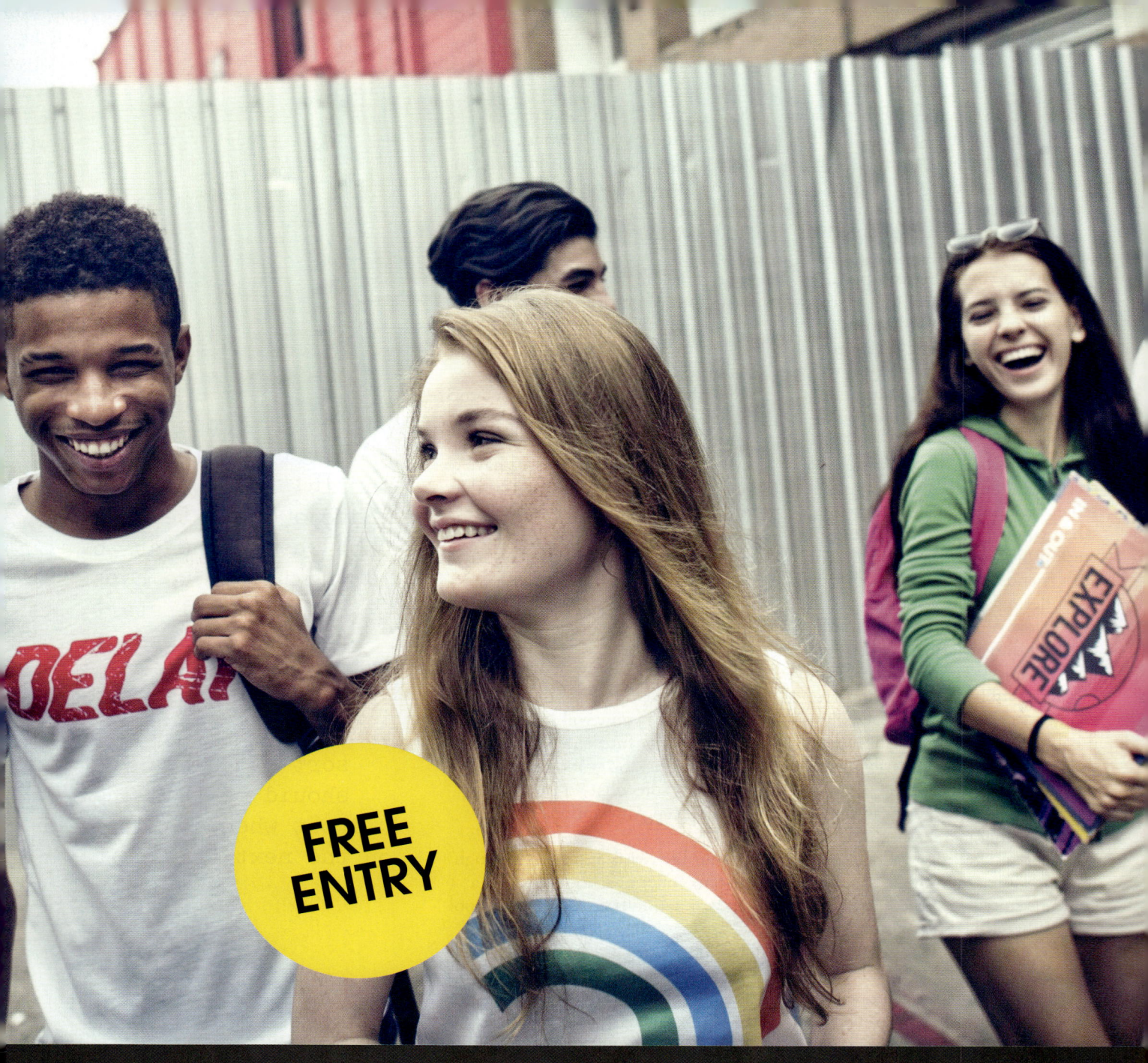

Meet the UK's top employers and universities

Meet over 100 exhibitors including*:

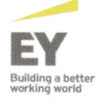

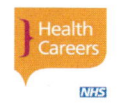

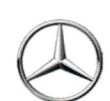

babcock · J.P.Morgan · EY Building a better working world · Health Careers NHS · VINCI Construction UK · Deloitte · ALDI · Mercedes

KPMG · Rolls-Royce · RSM · IBM · AON · NetworkRail · Boots · McDonald's

WB · Superdrug · HSBC · Schneider Electric · accenture High performance. Delivered. · hellmann Worldwide Logistics

What Career Live? in association with: The Telegraph · Apprenticeships

*Correct at time of print

What CAREER LIVE? What UNIVERSITY LIVE?

APPRENTICESHIP UNIVERSITY

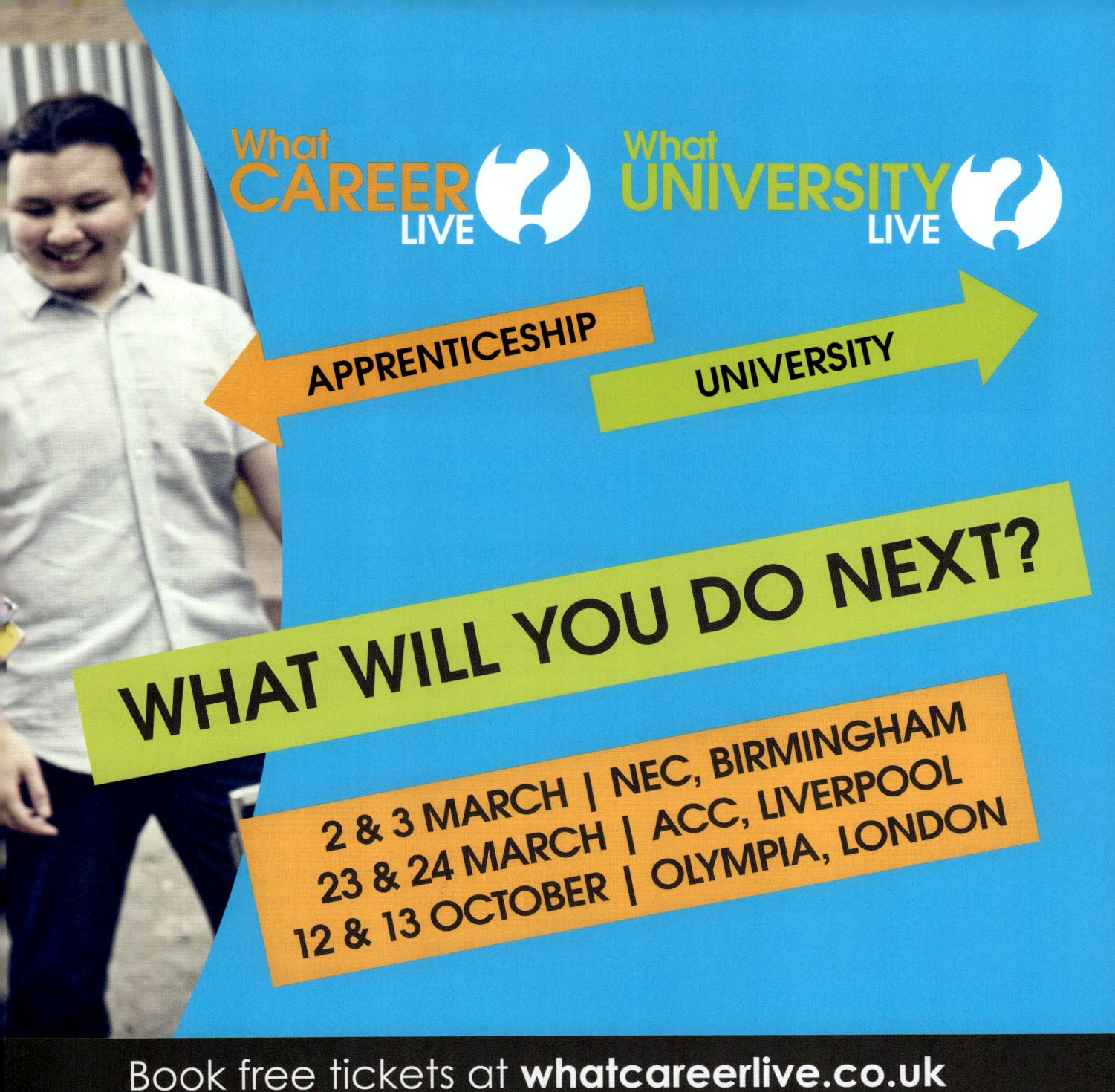

WHAT WILL YOU DO NEXT?

2 & 3 MARCH | NEC, BIRMINGHAM
23 & 24 MARCH | ACC, LIVERPOOL
12 & 13 OCTOBER | OLYMPIA, LONDON

Book free tickets at whatcareerlive.co.uk

UNIVERSITY OF BIRMINGHAM · University of Nottingham UK | CHINA | MALAYSIA · MANCHESTER 1824 · WARWICK THE UNIVERSITY OF WARWICK · University of BRISTOL · UNIVERSITY OF LEEDS

UNIVERSITY of DERBY · CITY UNIVERSITY LONDON · Coventry University · Keele University · The University of Law · Swansea University Prifysgol Abertawe

University of Roehampton London · Aston University Birmingham · UNIVERSITY OF Southampton · UNIVERSITY OF Hull · Teesside University

Brunel University London · Loughborough University · DE MONTFORT UNIVERSITY LEICESTER · UNIVERSITY OF LIVERPOOL · DISCOVER WITH PLYMOUTH UNIVERSITY · FULBRIGHT COMMISSION

f What Next?   @whatcareerlive   whatcareerlive

What University Live? in association with: UNIVERSITY OF LIVERPOOL

HEALTHCARE

Working within the healthcare sector can be rewarding for those of you who are interested in making a difference to people's health and well-being. If you want to have an impact on some of the most important issues that society is facing like the rise in obesity levels, cancer treatments and the increase in diabetes then this could be the sector for you.

Whether you like caring for people, carrying out research and testing, dealing with emergencies or problem solving, but above all, working with people, then you can find a role that will suit your skillset. The NHS is the largest employer in Europe, with over 1.3 million staff across the UK. There are also many private companies that work within the healthcare sector. You could find yourself working in various settings within the community; hospitals, care homes, GP surgeries, sports clubs, or laboratories.

There are many different jobs within the healthcare sector and here are just a few to get you thinking:

- Clinical Psychologist
- Healthcare Scientist
- Dental Health
- Nurse
- Optometrist
- Pharmacists
- Biomedical Scientist
- GP, Surgeon
- Carer
- Radiographer
- Sports and Exercise Scientist
- Paramedic

USEFUL RESOURCES

www.healthcareers.nhs.uk

www.careerprofiles.info.working-in-healthcare

We've picked a few interesting roles to explore in more detail...

CLINICAL PSYCHOLOGIST

The role of a Clinical Psychologist is improve the psychological wellbeing of their clients. They use different types of therapy to support their clients to make positive changes to their lives. Their clients might be experiencing different mental or physical issues such as anxiety, depression and eating disorders. To qualify as a clinical psychologist you need to study an undergraduate degree, followed by three years of postgraduate training. Gaining voluntary or paid work experience is essential to access this career.

BIOMEDICAL SCIENTIST

Biomedical scientists work to diagnose disease and evaluate the effectiveness of treatment through the analysis of fluids and tissue samples from patients. They may work on understanding medical conditions, such as cancer, diabetes, AIDS and malaria. Most people who go into biomedical science have a relevant degree, and each individual needs to be registered with the Health and Care Professions Council. However, it is possible to enter the career with A-Levels and your employer will support you to study for a degree part time.

SOCIAL CARER

Care workers are the front line staff who work with all types of people who need care and support. They are responsible for the individuals' overall comfort and wellbeing and they help people who need care and support to live as independently as possible. You don't need formal qualifications to be a carer and there will be plenty of opportunities to acquire more skills, training and qualifications depending on how far you want to take your career in the sector.

OPTOMETRIST

Optometry is the care of eyes and vision, identifying injuries and diseases as well as prescribing glasses and contact lenses. Optometrists also work with other health professionals to help care for patients' general health. For example, conditions like diabetes can affect the eyes, and optometrists can both help to manage the resulting problems and will sometimes identify the diabetes in the first place. In order to qualify as an optometrist you need to study an Optometry degree which is offered at 11 universities across the UK.

MEDICAL APPLICANTS

Medicine is an incredibly rewarding and respected career. Although it is exciting and dynamic it is ultimately about helping people, about being willing to put someone else's needs first and doing all that you can to improve their health and wellbeing.

It is far from an easy option – it takes years of study and hard work, but if you want to push yourself and also have a passion to improve people's lives, it could be the right thing for you.

Medicine is a challenging career, but the two most important things you must have to succeed are an enquiring mind and the ability to relate to people as individuals, each with their own health needs. Very few areas of work can match the variety of medicine – it will confront you with something new every day. The profession is also concerned with integrity and is committed to uphold a number of timeless values.

APPLYING TO MEDICAL SCHOOL

Undergraduate medicine courses last approximately five years and the course can vary significantly depending on which university you attend. Some universities offer Problem Based Learning (PBL) course which allows students to set their own learning goals and working through various clinical problems with the help of an experienced tutor. This is becoming a very popular form of teaching and is something you should think about when selecting your university. Work experience is a really important part of the medical profession and it is essential to try and get as much experience under your belt before you reach medical school. Although it is often difficult to find work experience opportunities in hospitals, there are plenty of alternatives that demonstrate your compassion and ability to care for others e.g. shadowing a district nurse, care homes or centres for the homeless. Universities now require students to take aptitude tests such as the UKCAT and BMAT. These tests help support your application and they are used in conjunction with your personal statement and A-Level grades.

MEDICAL SCHOOL AND BEYOND

After graduation from medical school, doctors undertake a clinical apprenticeship and learning is undertaken while actually doing the job. The apprenticeship begins at the foundation house officer grade and continues until you become a consultant or a GP. It is also important to remember that doctors have to update their knowledge and skills throughout their career.

To a certain extent, doctors are able to choose in which area of medicine they practise. Within the practice of medicine there are over 60 different specialities, each with their own particular characteristics. For example, community-based doctors like GPs have daily face-to-face contact with patients, while other doctors might focus on scientific research that involves less patient contact. Your medical training will give you the opportunity to discover which appeals to you most and can involve studying abroad. Although the majority of doctors work within the NHS, opportunities exist in other settings, such as the armed forces, the Home Office, working as a police surgeon or as a prison doctor, and many others. In your future career you will have good job security and further opportunities to work in another country. Medicine can take you wherever you want to go.

Once you become a doctor you will need to register with the General Medical Council (GMC) and are strongly advised to acquire medical insurance. Most doctors also become members of the British Medical Association (BMA).

GETTING INTO MEDICAL SCHOOL

We all know it's a challenge, with ratios in excess of ten applicants per place. So given the high level of competition, what is it that makes you "stand out from the crowd" in applying for medicine?

> The quick and pedantic answer is "a poor quality application"; with so many highly qualified, well-prepared and enthusiastic applicants it's far easier to spot the poor quality outlier from amongst the wealth of excellence. So rather than attempt the impossible in offering any sure-fire route to success, I'll instead offer broader guidance that helps you engage with the deeper thinking at play in selecting tomorrow's doctors.

MOTIVATION

All medical schools are looking for applicants with enthusiasm – individuals who are genuinely motivated by the idea of working in medicine. The challenge for you is to critically reflect on this motivation. All too often applicants have told me in interviews that they have "wanted to be a doctor ever since they were five", so let's critically reflect on that statement – as a five-year-old, how well informed were you of what it meant to be a doctor? How aware were you of your abilities and your limitations? When I was five I wanted to be an astronaut, but by the time I was ten I'd grown out of it. As an individual you need to actively challenge your motivation through constructive critique; always be prepared to step out of yourself and ask an uncomfortable question. This is what will help you reach that deeper level of understanding and engagement.

WORK EXPERIENCE

The challenge here is to get out of the 'tick-box' mentality, not to treat work experience as a test to complete, but as an opportunity to learn. You need a good understanding of what makes you tick; your strengths and, very importantly, your weaknesses (aka your opportunities for growth). A useful approach is to think of work experience (and voluntary experience, and life experience) as a chance to build evidence, both to help confirm your thoughts and to convince a medical school of your suitability. Identify the key skills that are needed to be a doctor – such as communication, empathy and integrity – and identify examples from your own life where you have demonstrated those skills. And genuinely do not be afraid to engage with your weaknesses – it is far healthier to have a mentality that recognises "failure" as an opportunity to learn, rather than something to be ashamed of.

There are many different types of experience out there, ranging from shadowing a consultant in a hospital right through to working in your local shop. You might assume that the clinical experience is preferable, but not if you fail to demonstrate learning from it. Medical schools also recognise that access to clinical placements is not equitable (not everyone has an aunt or a neighbour who can help secure a place), so they consider the full breadth of potential experience, and consider your reflections on experience just as much, if not more so, than the actual experience itself. The key is to focus on opportunities to learn and opportunities to demonstrate the active application of key skills – take a look at www.tasteofmedicine.com for an in-depth exploration of the full range of potential experiences, recognising that all types of experience offer an opportunity to develop and to reflect.

CORE SKILLS vs SPECIFIC KNOWLEDGE

As a medical student you will spend many years studying at university, taught by experts in their field who will help you develop the medical knowledge you need to be successful as a doctor. Concurrently these experts will facilitate the development of your core skills (noting that is different to being 'taught'). That medical knowledge is not something expected of you before you start, but you are expected to be able to demonstrate and engage with the core underlying skills. It is important to recognise the differences between "knowing facts" and "knowing how to apply facts", and that is where demonstrating a propensity in core skills, such as empathy, resilience, insight and team working, will be of real value.

KEEPING PERSPECTIVE

Too easily the process of applying for medical school becomes a race, an all-encompassing focal point to your life. Yes, it is important, and yes you need to devote time and attention to it, but to do so at the expense of other priorities can be damaging. It may be hard to read, but "don't be in a rush to be a doctor". As one of the very few genuine life-long careers left in modern society, you can realistically expect still to be working as a doctor when you retire. Always keep in mind other routes, like clinical transfer from Biomedical Science, graduate entry, or joining medicine as a career change.

The other key perspective not to lose sight of is who you are – your friends, your family and your life. Focussing on academic work at the expense of your social life can hinder your application. You may find that by spending your days in the library you're able to secure excellent grades, but at what cost? Key skills of empathy, integrity, communication and insight can't be easily learnt from a book. It's engaging with life that helps you develop: meeting new people; experiencing new activities; and embracing what the world has to offer. So never underestimate the importance of maintaining a life/work balance, ensuring you fully engage with relaxing, recuperating and enjoying life.

CONCLUSIONS

DON'T BE IN A RUSH
If you want to be a doctor then go for it, but don't be hard on yourself if you don't get in first time. Keep in mind the alternatives, both in terms of related careers and other routes into medical training.

FOCUS ON THE CORE SKILLS
You are not expected to be an expert in all things medical, but you are expected to have the underlying skills and abilities necessary to develop as a medical student and a doctor. Focus on the core skills and link these to the experiences you've had.

KEEP PERSPECTIVE
Applying for medicine can dominate your life and become an urgent priority. But don't let the 'urgent' distract you from what is 'important' – a balance that allows you to enjoy life, develop as a human being, and achieve success in the widest sense of the word.

Dr Kenton Lewis MBE

Dr Kenton Lewis MBE (www.kentonlewis.co.uk) is an independent education consultant, executive coach and mediator. He has guided and advised thousands of students, having worked at the University of Oxford, the University of Bristol and, for ten years, running Student Recruitment at St George's, University of London.

ALTERNATIVE ROUTES INTO MEDICINE

Medicine is by far the UK's most popular undergraduate course, and with over 20,000 applicants for 7,500 places, many applicants will not get a place. In the face of such fierce competition, all budding medics should have a plan B in place, just in case your application isn't successful. If your application to medical school has been unsuccessful, or you missed the required grades on results day, there are three different pathways available to you.

1. THE GRADUATE ENTRY PROGRAMME

The Graduate Entry Programme (GEP) is a four year qualification which can be completed after graduating from university with a scientific degree. If you gain a 2:1 or higher in a subject such as Biomedical Sciences, Biochemistry and Natural Sciences then you would be eligible to apply for the GEP.

If you achieve less than 2:1 or your undergraduate degree was not in a scientific subject then you will need to take the Access to Medicine course prior to starting the GEP. These courses are primarily run by further education colleges, but there are a handful of universities who also offer the course.

It is important to bear in mind that some medical schools do accept students on their GEP courses without the Access to Medicine qualification, so it would be advisable to check on the information on the UCAS website or the individual university websites.

2. OTHER RELATED COURSES

There are several other careers related to medicine for which you may be suitable, and which will provide a very rewarding career path. These include:

- Clinical Psychologist
- Healthcare Scientist
- Dental Health
- Nurse
- Optometrist
- Pharmacists
- Radiographer
- Physiotherapist
- Sports and Exercise Scientist
- Paramedic

This is not an exhaustive list, and there are many more careers worth investigating. Many of these professions require a very similar set of skills to that of a doctor and can be equally rewarding.

3. RETAKING & REAPPLYING

If you did not achieve the grades that you wanted, it is possible to take a year out to retake your exams and reapply to medical schools. It is common for universities to accept re-takes, but they may increase their standard offer so it is important to check this. If you did not secure an offer at a medical school but achieved outstanding results in your exams you might be interested in taking a gap year and reapplying. The main advantage with this is that you can apply with your actual grades rather than predicted. When reapplying, we advise you to look back over your UCAS form and personal statement and look at ways to improve your application. The universities will want to know what you have done in your year out to make yourself a more attractive candidate. It would be very helpful if you could combine your year out with a relevant part-time job within the healthcare sector, as this would dramatically improve your personal statement and your chances of securing a place.

MY EXPERIENCE

Andrew Durnford
Neurosurgery Doctor at University Hospital Southampton

"My day-to-day tasks vary from treating acutely unwell patients including performing emergency operations, as well as seeing patients in clinic and managing conditions affecting the brain and spine, often with surgery. There are also opportunities to undertake medical research and potentially change the future treatment of patients. My role requires good relationships with many different colleagues in a hospital, including x-ray doctors to help make correct diagnoses and also those involved in rehabilitation of patients following surgery, such as physiotherapists.

As a trainee surgeon I am paid a full salary. Although medical training can take many years, the continual learning and challenges represent one of the most enjoyable aspects of the job. I enjoy surgery as it is practical and requires excellent problem solving, judgement and communication skills, to enable you to help and care for people of all different ages and backgrounds. I went to a local comprehensive school and studied A-Levels and then studied at Oxford University and Birmingham University before becoming a junior doctor.

Becoming a doctor involves getting good grades at A-Level then studying medicine at university typically for 5 years. You then start as a full-time junior doctor working for two years in a hospital before choosing to pursue a career often either as a GP or hospital doctor within many diverse branches of medicine including surgery. Opportunities also exist to work abroad in both developed and developing countries, in the armed forces or in academic research at universities allied to NHS hospitals."

Amanda Williamson
Clinical Audit and Effectiveness Manager at a District General Hospital

"I manage a team of 14 people who undertake a number of roles linked to governance. This means we take the local trust's annual audit plan for the hospital and ensure it is completed each year. We also help format clinical policies, procedures, and guidelines for clinicians and check them through an approval process. I review any guidance from external bodies (such as the National Institute for Health and Care Excellence or the National Confidential Enquires into Patient Outcome and Death) that is published and, if relevant to our trust, I send out to clinicians to determine if the Trust already complies to the recommendations or if we need to make any changes to ensure we meet them. The team also supports the NHS National Patient Surveys for our trust and I undertake monthly analysis of patient feedback, escalating any concerns to senior nurses and identifying areas for improvement to patient experience whilst they're in the hospital. Every day is different!

You could definitely say I 'fell' into this role. I originally trained as a nurse and a midwife and worked in clinical practice for a number of years. I worked part time as a midwife for a few years and during that time I undertook a bachelor's degree in Law followed by a master's degree in Family Law and Policy. Following this, I undertook a teaching role at a university for a number of years before returning to the NHS and clinical practice where I commenced my current role.

The best thing about my role is knowing that my job and my team helps to improve patient outcomes and patient experience in the hospital. I like being up to date with current clinical practice and national recommendations, I am always learning something new. The most challenging part of the role is trying to get some people to engage with us - we need excellent communication and diplomatic skills! Although this is quite a specialist role, you could approach it from a number of different ways. Some of my team have worked in clinical practice as nurses, some have undertaken degrees such as Applied Pyschology or English, and others have worked in administration. I think my top tip for getting into something similar would be to do a degree or course in something you enjoy and gain NHS experience working with people."

FINANCE

Finance is a broad term that covers a wide range of jobs to do with money, including banking, insurance, investment, and lots more. There is such a wide range of roles within the sector that there really is a job for everyone, you just have to research to find out what suits you - from behind the scenes research, to on the trading floor, working with huge corporations to helping a family budget.

To succeed in this sector you will need to be able to communicate well and be comfortable talking to people from across all levels. You'll need to be an effective negotiator and able to work well under pressure. Working in finance can mean working long hours in a fast-paced environment so it particularly suits people who are highly motivated and determined. Contrary to popular belief you do not need to be a mathematical genius to succeed!

There are many different roles within this sector, and here are just a few to get you thinking:

- Accountant
- Business Analyst
- External Auditor
- Financial Analyst
- Tax, Finance Director
- Mortgage Broker
- Risk Manager
- Actuary
- Credit Analyst
- Asset Manager
- Hedge Fund Manager
- Broker
- Investment Manager

USEFUL RESOURCES

www.careers-in-finance.com
www.prospects.ac.uk
www.investopedia.com

We've picked a few interesting roles to explore in more detail...

ACCOUNTANCY
Accountants generally work with the financial side of a business and interpret the figures and advise accordingly. There are many different kinds of accounting: tax, audit, government, bookkeeper and forensic (detecting fraud).

FINANCIAL SERVICES AND INSURANCE
If you like the idea of helping people plan their futures, then this area could be for you. By providing expert advice (gathered through research with doctors, lawyers, and fire officers to name but a few to assess risk) you can help families save money through insurance, mortgages and carefully financial planning, and resolve claims against insurance companies.

BANKING
The biggest employers in the finance sector, these enable individuals and businesses to manage their money and access products such as loans, both in the UK and overseas. The term covers a huge range of jobs, from the high street banks you probably walk past every day, to the financial institutions that you hear about in the news.

INVESTMENT MANAGEMENT
Your job here would involve researching funds and making an educated guess on their likely performance. You would advise asset managers, and depending on the area you specialise in you could be including trading and stockbroking, performance measurement, investment support, risk assessment and data management.

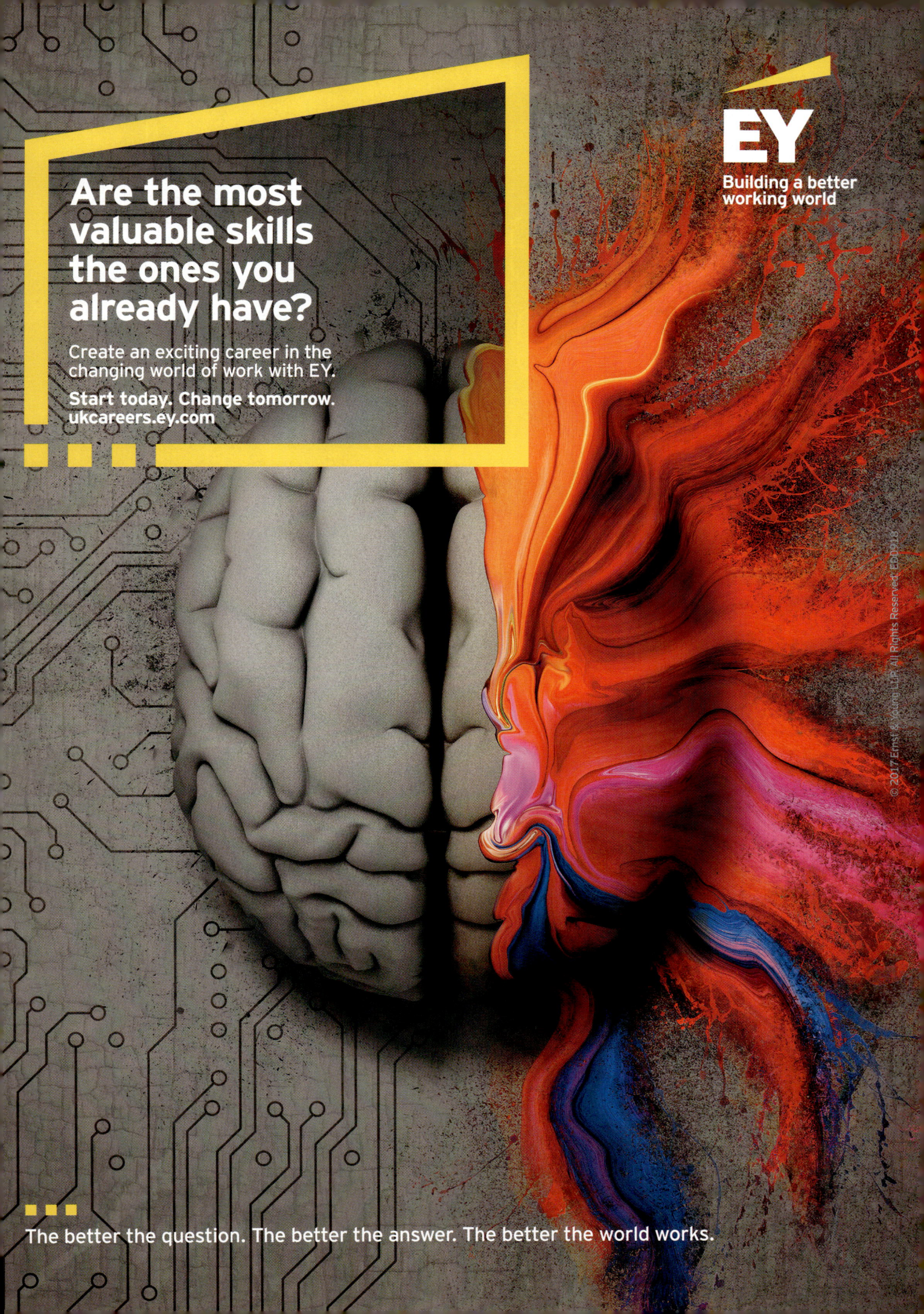

Are the most valuable skills the ones you already have?

Create an exciting career in the changing world of work with EY.

Start today. Change tomorrow.
ukcareers.ey.com

EY
Building a better working world

The better the question. The better the answer. The better the world works.

KPMG

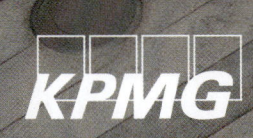

Experience can be the greatest teacher

**Apprenticeship Programmes
Autumn 2018**

KPMG360°
KPMG360° Digital

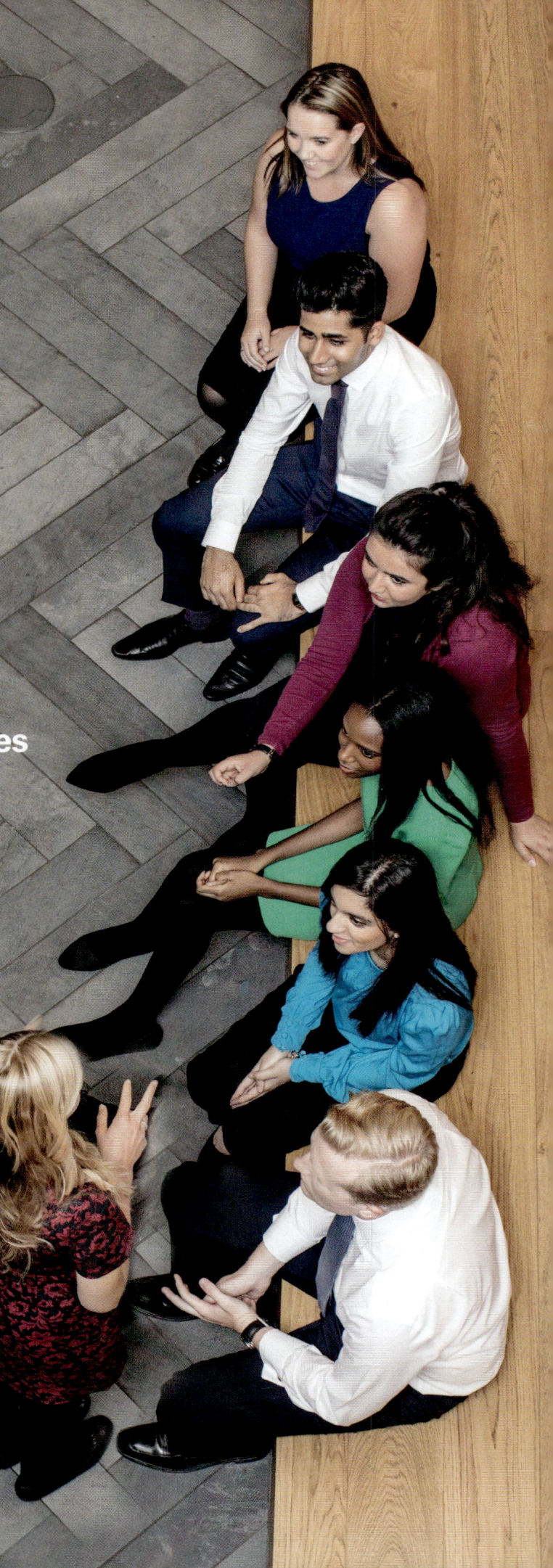

Are you ready to realise your potential?

As a KPMG apprentice, we'll invest in you from day one. You'll receive great benefits, structured training and an exceptional level of support – we want to inspire you to be your best.

Why do an apprenticeship?

Instead of following the traditional university route, you'll earn while you learn. Whilst exploring our business, you'll also gain the skills and experience needed to become a truly accomplished professional.

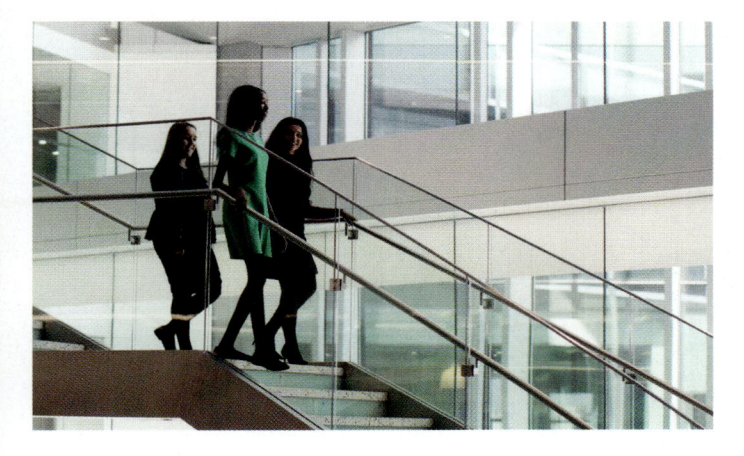

How do I apply?

At KPMG, we come from diverse backgrounds and our behaviours unite us. Our decision to offer you a place will be based on a well-rounded view. Taking several factors into account, we'll be looking at three key areas: your academic results, experiences and interests – and of course, how you perform in our exercises.

Which programmes do we have to offer you?

We have two Apprenticeship Programmes available:

KPMG360° gives you the chance to join KPMG and work with some of the best and brightest in the business world. Importantly, it includes a foundation year that's specifically designed so you can experience all areas of the business before you choose a specialist area and gain a professional qualification.

KPMG360° Digital is a new four-year Apprenticeship Programme that combines academic study with practical work experience. At the same time, you'll also study for a BSc degree in Digital and Technology Solutions with our training provider, BPP University.

Our Deal – what benefits do KPMG offer you?

As an apprentice, you're an important part of the future of our business, so we'll reward your contribution in a number of ways. In addition to the exclusive KPMG 'Our Deal' benefits, you'll also receive: 25 days holiday, a competitive salary, pension options and a travel season ticket loan. In addition you'll also receive an extra day off on your birthday, lunch allowance, financial support towards gaining professional qualifications and study leave.

Hear from a KPMG apprentice

Ann-Marie started the KPMG360o Programme after finishing her A-levels. "Working at a firm with such a big reputation opens so many opportunities. The fact that I am earning money instead of being in university and taking on debt means I have never regretted my decision not to go to university." Hear more from Ann-Marie here: kpmgcareers.co.uk/ann-marie

Top tips for applying

At KPMG we are looking for 9 behavioural capabilities. These capabilities are what you will be assessed on throughout the recruitment process. You should research the behavioural capabilities, KPMG values and the KPMG360o programme itself. Overall, try to be yourself and enjoy the experience!

Don't forget to follow us on Facebook, Twitter and Instagram to hear the latest from us too!

Curious?

Whichever programme you choose, you'll be making a great start to your career. You'll gain a thorough understanding of how businesses work, and develop the skills to help build a successful and fulfilling career at KPMG.

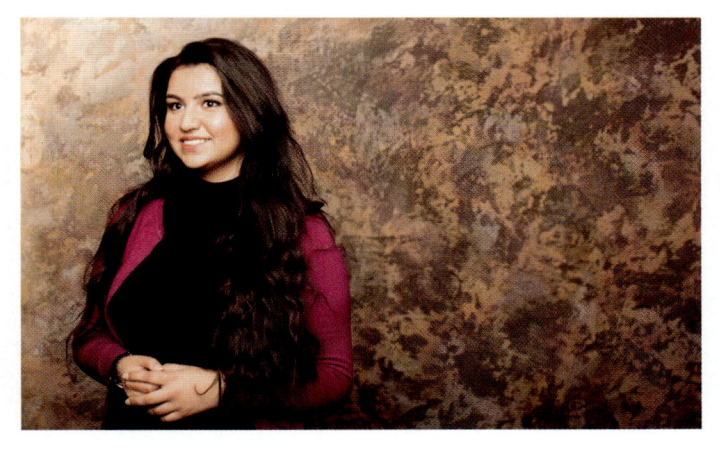

Find out more about what we can offer you and apply today by visiting our careers site here:
kpmgcareers.co.uk/apprenticeships

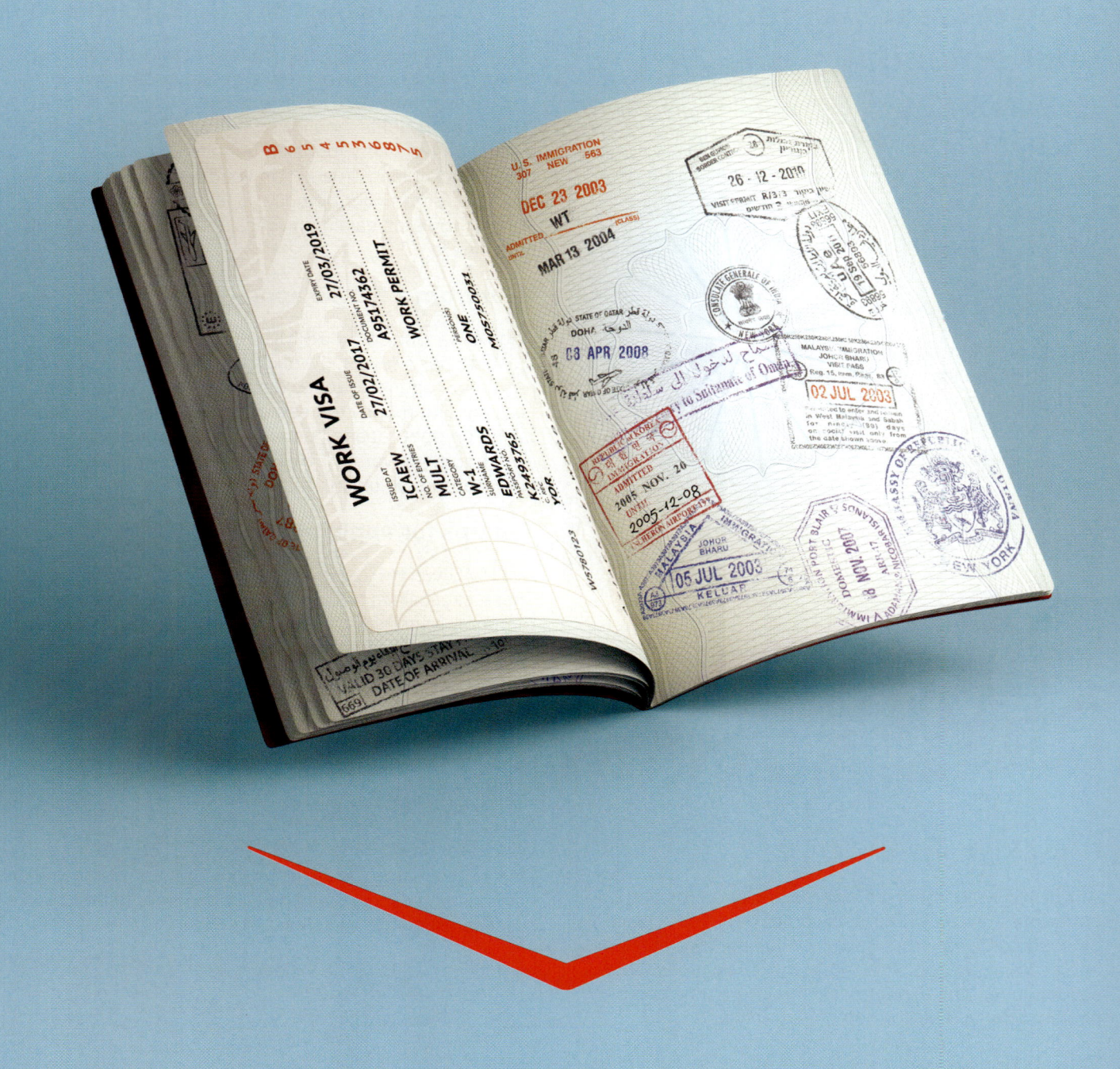

Go places. Become an ICAEW Chartered Accountant.

Take your career to more destinations than you'd imagine as an ICAEW Chartered Accountant. With a focus on innovative thinking, ethics and leadership, you'll become a strategic business leader. And because ICAEW Chartered Accountancy is recognised and respected in 154 countries worldwide, you really can go places.

Learn more at **icaew.com/careers**

ICAEW

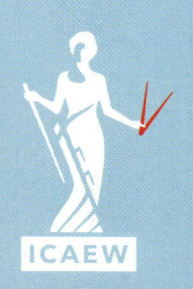

More rewarding

More success

AVERAGE GLOBAL SALARY
£49.9K
0-2 YEARS POST QUALIFICATION

FIRST TIME PASS RATE IS
79%
FOR ICAEW STUDENTS

98
OF THE WORLD'S 100 GLOBAL LEADING BRANDS EMPLOY ICAEW CHARTERED ACCOUNTANTS

ICAEW HAS 147,000 MEMBERS
147,000
WORKING IN 154 COUNTRIES

ICAEW ACCOUNTANTS ARE ON
78 OF THE BOARDS
OF FTSE 100 COMPANIES

More respected

More global

More prestigious

ICAEW.
More than you'd imagine.

LAW

If you want a career that will keep your mind engaged, law could be a great choice. Whichever route you take, you will need to have an avid interest in the law as it is intellectually demanding.

Every aspect of our society is governed by law and accordingly there are all kinds of lawyers. Whatever your interests, there will be an area of law governing it and legal professionals practicing it. If you feel passionately about human rights or international politics, a career in public or European law may await you. If you find yourself attracted to business and commerce, you might find a perfect home in one of the big City firms. If you find yourself waiting with bated breath for the new edition of 'Heat' to fall through your letterbox, Defamation and Media Law could be the area for you. The rewards of a career in law are as varied as the different areas of practice. Corporate law in a large firm will bring with it a secure and hefty salary. Criminal law may provide the satisfaction of preserving an innocent person's liberty or ensuring that the guilty are brought to account.

Many lawyers would say that the main attraction of working in the law is the intellectual challenge it presents. The law is evolving all the time. Textbooks are changed and revised constantly, as new concepts come to light and new rights are recognised. This means that lawyers in all fields are always innovating and adapting to new circumstances.

You DO NOT need to study law at university to become a lawyer. Thinking that studying law is a must is the most common misconception that students have about a legal career. Whether you want to work as a legal executive, city lawyer, in family law, at an international firm, as an in-house lawyer or as a barrister for a chamber, there are a number of routes in, and studying law as an undergraduate student at university is not the only one. In fact some law firms prefer students who have broader interests and have studied something other than law. There are three main routes into law, outlined here:

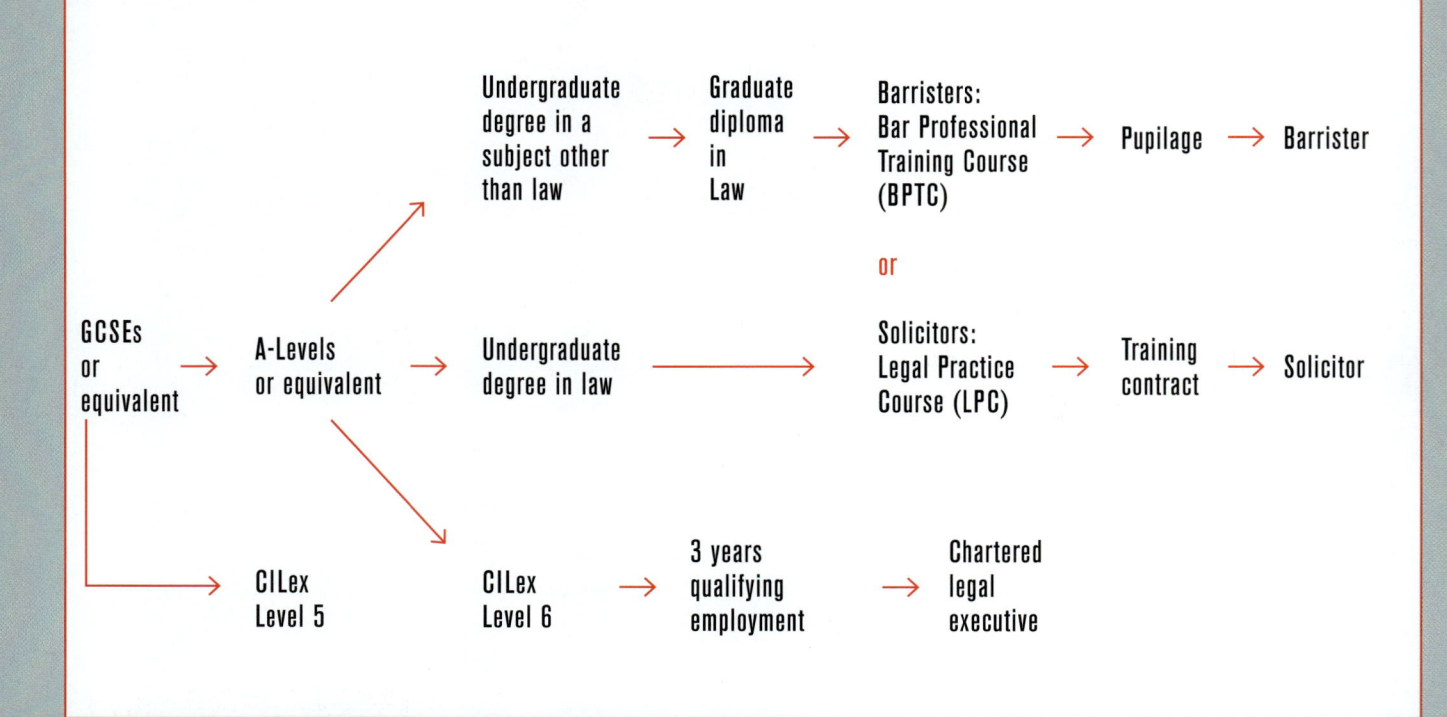

GCSEs or equivalent → A-Levels or equivalent → Undergraduate degree in a subject other than law → Graduate diploma in Law → Barristers: Bar Professional Training Course (BPTC) → Pupilage → Barrister

or

A-Levels or equivalent → Undergraduate degree in law → Solicitors: Legal Practice Course (LPC) → Training contract → Solicitor

GCSEs or equivalent → CILex Level 5 → CILex Level 6 → 3 years qualifying employment → Chartered legal executive

~~SUCCESS~~ SUPPORT BREEDS SUCCESS

We place a huge emphasis on providing the right support and training so you can truly fulfil your potential.

That's why, at Gowling WLG, you'll get the training and support you need to become a dynamic, well-rounded lawyer, and you'll work alongside inspirational colleagues who are at the top of their field. Best of all, you'll begin your career at the only law firm to appear in the Great Place to Work UK 2017 rankings.

Join us – to find out more and apply today go to:
gowlingwlgcareers.co.uk

APPRENTICSHIP OPPORTUNITIES
An international law firm that's ambitious for your success

GOWLING WLG

Gowling WLG (UK) LLP is a member of Gowling WLG, an international law firm which consists of independent and autonomous entities providing services around the world. Our structure is explained in more detail at www.gowlingwlg.com/legal

There are many different roles within this sector, and here are just a few to get you thinking:

```
Solicitor
In-house Lawyer
Barrister
Legal Executive
Judge
Paralegal
Researcher for the Law Commission
Court Usher
Conveyancer
Legal Secretary
```

USEFUL RESOURCES

l2b.thelawyer.com
www.cilex.org.uk
www.lawsociety.org.uk
www.barcouncil.org.uk
www.theiop.org

We've picked a few interesting roles to explore in more detail…

COURT USHER
A court usher is a position in a law court. You will need to escort participants to the courtroom, check that witnesses, defendants and lawyers are all present, direct the taking of oaths, correctly label evidence and handle it carefully where required, and ensure the secure transaction of legal documents within the courtroom and deciding the order of cases. You'll need to have strong people skills to deal with every member of the court room.

LEGAL SECRETARY
Legal secretaries are an essential part of all legal practices, and this career oath can be an excellent way to embark on a legal career without committing to further study. If you enjoy the work that you do, you can upskill as you go along, gaining law qualifications while you work.

CONVEYANCER
A licensed conveyancer is someone who deals specifically with property transactions, so you would only need to gain the knowledge and qualifications for this specific area of law, i.e. the buying and selling of domestic and commercial properties. This qualification can be gained without going to university, so you avoid racking up debt.

PARALEGAL
A paralegal is a person qualified through education and training to perform substantive legal work that requires knowledge of the law and procedures but who is not a qualified solicitor or barrister, although their work does overlap. They usually specialise in just one specific area of law and become an expert in it.

Paralegal job roles vary depending on where you work and the experience and qualifications you have, you could work for a huge firm being part of a large team, or at a high street solicitor assisting on smaller contracts. Work can range from administrative and legal secretarial tasks to undertaking research and providing legal information to clients. You will need to have excellent communication skills to deal with clients from a wide range of backgrounds, and manage your time well to meet deadlines.

It is common for a budding solicitor to work as a paralegal for a year or two while they apply for training contracts.

SOLICITOR
To succeed as a solicitor, you need to be determined and willing to work hard. It will take at least three years to train if you are a law graduate, at least four years if you are a non-law graduate and at least six years if you are not a graduate. It is intellectually challenging, and there are a wide range of areas you can specialise in, including family law, criminal law, banking and finance law and corporate law, to name a few.

JUDGE
Judges are the public officers who decide cases in a law court, and you will probably have seen them portrayed in film and television. They preside over court proceedings, sometimes as part of a panel. Judges are only appointed by the Judicial Appointments Commission after practicing law for a number of years, you cannot train to be a judge straight from school or university.

BRIGHT SPARKS

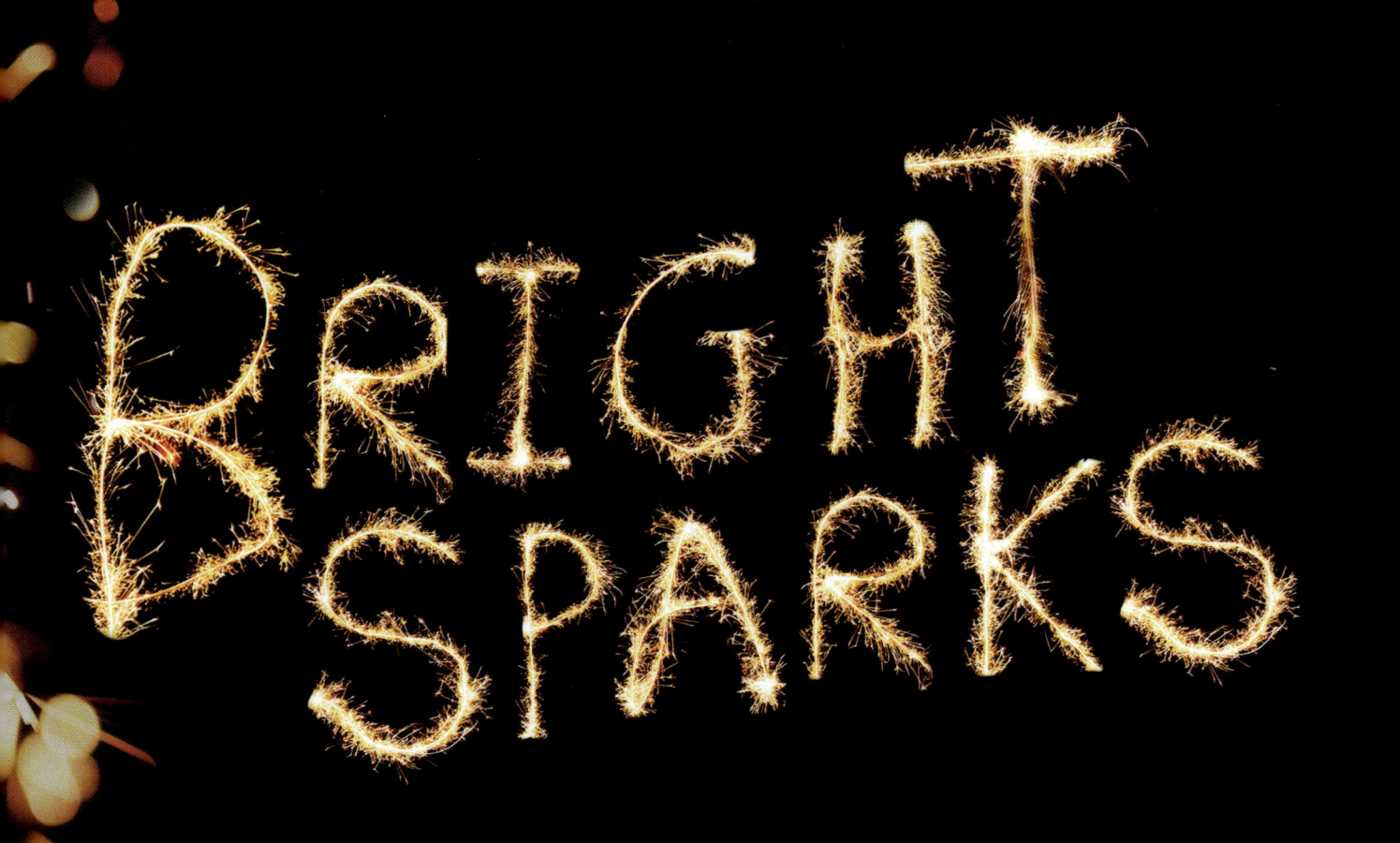

Giving young talent the chance to shine

Work experience with an international law firm for talented year 12 students

If you're thinking of a career in Law, Marketing, HR, Finance or IT, this is the perfect place to start. A chance to develop your personal and professional skills, brush up on your CV and interview techniques, get some real-world experience and find where your strengths and interests lie.

For full details and to download an application form visit:
www.shlegal.com/graduate/brightsparks

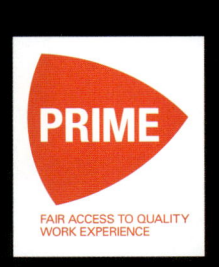

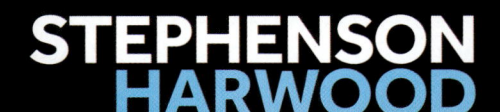

PRIME — FAIR ACCESS TO QUALITY WORK EXPERIENCE

STEPHENSON HARWOOD

LAW INTERVIEW

WHAT DO YOU LIKE MOST ABOUT BEING A LAWYER?

"I have really enjoyed being part of a team working on a deal which makes the papers or gets discussed on TV. Although small in the context of a wider transaction, the tasks for trainees on these high-profile matters are often pivotal to their success or failure (for example, a research note into a specifically problematic legal area). That feeling of accomplishment, knowing that your hard work was an important component in the successful completion of a deal or winning of a case, is something which definitely motivates me to actually get up when my alarm goes every morning!"

"I really enjoy working with lots of different people. Also, it's great to be given different tasks and varying levels of responsibility. With each task I'm given, I get to be involved in a different aspect of the firm's practice and this means that I always maintain an interest in what I am doing. For example, when working on a pitch to a potential client I am helping with business development, whereas, when drafting documents for a live deal, I'm helping the team prepare the many legal documents that we're under pressure to put in place for the deal to close."

ARE THERE ANY ASPECTS YOU DON'T LIKE SO MUCH?

"In the midst of all the excitement, the hours can be occasionally long depending on client expectations and workload. This is especially challenging when I want to rush home to watch a football game in the evening."

"As a trainee you often have to carry out various administrative tasks (i.e. anything from copy checking to creating bundles of documents). However, you start to realise that everyone who is more senior than you has been through this process and this kind of work is a stepping-stone to the more rewarding and stimulating work. I think it's good to take pride in every piece of work you do as this starts to make even the least interesting jobs more satisfying."

WHAT ADVICE WOULD YOU GIVE THE READERS THINKING OF GOING INTO A LEGAL CAREER?

"The legal profession is a broad one, filled with variety. My advice is to research which aspect of law interests you most, which is usually determined by which aspect of life interests you most! For example, you can go into sports law, family law, media law or public law. The possibilities are endless. Once you have identified which area of law interests you, try and get some work experience at a firm which specialises in that type of work. That way, you'll have a taste of life in practice and you will stand out from the crowd should you decide to pursue a legal career."

"It is worth trying to get some work experience under your belt. Even if it is just for a couple of days, having it on your CV will demonstrate that you have a genuine interest in a career in law."

"Just work as hard as you can, both academically and by getting involved in extra-curricular activities. I think it is really important to gain as much varied experience as possible. I am so happy to be working at an international law firm, and despite the endless hours of revision, essay writing, every minute has proved worthwhile. I would recommend law to anyone committed enough to put the hours in."

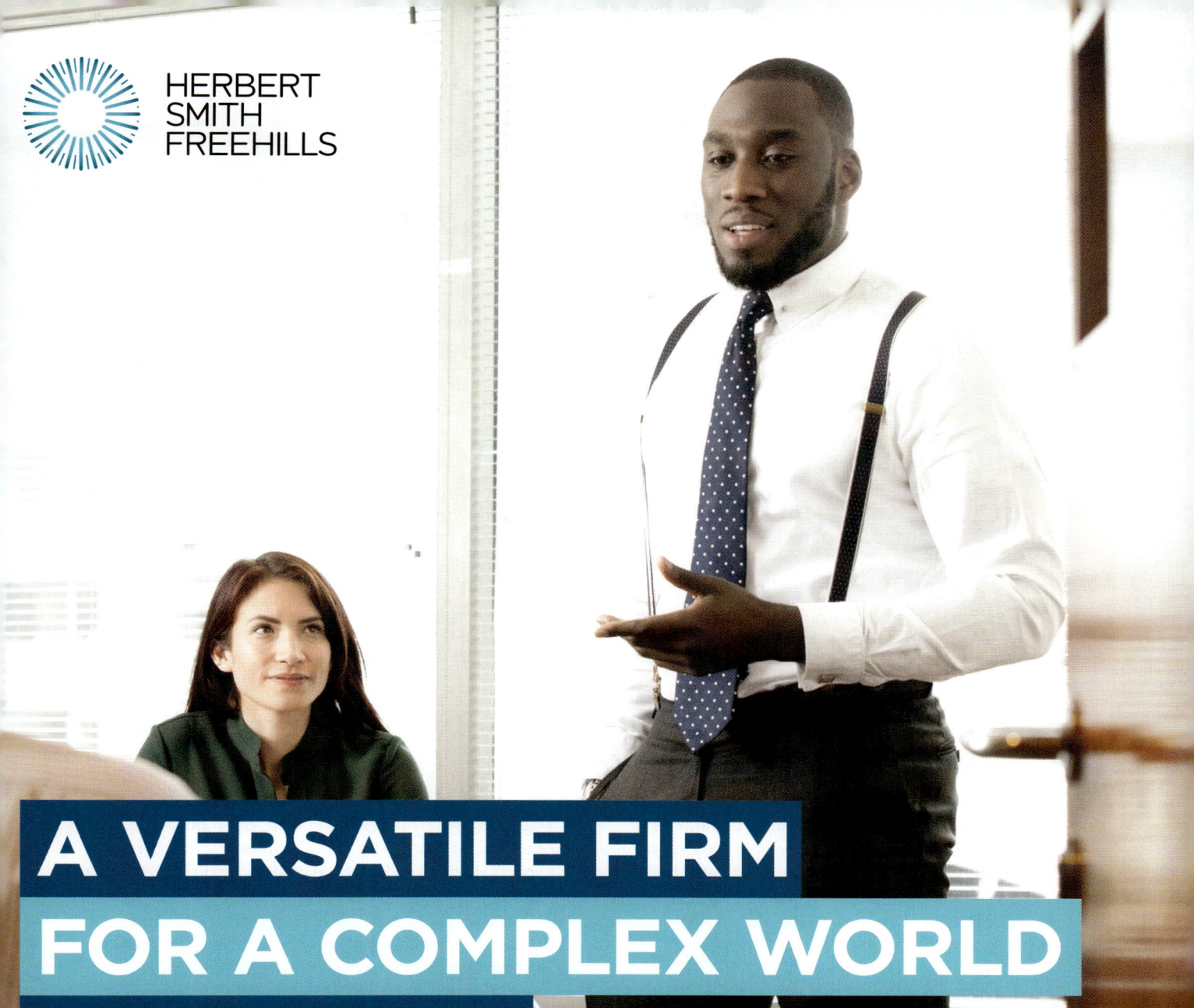

HERBERT SMITH FREEHILLS

A VERSATILE FIRM FOR A COMPLEX WORLD
BE A PART OF EVERYTHING

JOIN A TEAM WITH GLOBAL IMPACT

Different backgrounds. Progressive thinking. Global perspectives. At Herbert Smith Freehills we recognise and value all the differences that make each of us unique. By embracing a diversity of views and experience, we provide our clients with the most innovative advice. Inclusivity and diversity doesn't just mean a better place to work, it makes us more successful as a firm.

HOW TO APPLY

1. COMPLETE AN APPLICATION FORM
2. TAKE AN ONLINE VERBAL REASONING TEST
3. COME TO OUR ASSESSMENT CENTRE

FACTS

- 26 OFFICES GLOBALLY
- 220 INTERNATIONAL SECONDMENTS
- £44k IN FIRST YEAR

ROLES

- FIRST YEAR WORKSHOPS
- VACATION SCHEMES
- TRAINING CONTRACTS

SEARCH **HSF GRADUATES**

HOW TO BECOME A BARRISTER

Barristers provide specialist legal advice and represent their clients in courts and tribunals. Their work is intellectually challenging in an intense and demanding professional environment. It can also be a very rewarding career. Barristers' work varies considerably depending on the area of law they practise in and their seniority.

TYPICALLY, BARRISTERS DO SOME OR ALL OF THE FOLLOWING:

- Advise clients on the law and the strength of their legal case.
- Hold 'conferences' with clients to discuss taking their case forward and giving them legal advice.
- Represent clients in court. This can include presenting the case, cross-examining witnesses, summing up all relevant material and giving reasons why the court should support the case.
- Negotiate settlements with the other side.

Most barristers are self-employed and work in chambers, although approximately 20% are at the 'employed Bar' and work for an employer, an industry, commerce or central or local government for example the Crown Prosecution Service. The role of an employed barrister can vary greatly depending on their employer. The majority will work in specialist legal departments advising only the organisation they work for.

Self-employed barristers work in offices called chambers that they probably share with other barristers. On completion of their training, barristers apply for a permanent position, called tenancy, in a set of a chambers.

Students are expected to demonstrate the following skills in order to both qualify as a barrister and succeed in the competitive professional and business world:

- Academic ability (at least a 2:1 at degree level)
- Outstanding communication skills
- An ability to absorb and analyse complex information, often very quickly
- Numeracy skills
- Interpersonal skills
- Good judgement
- A high level of self-motivation
- Commitment to continuing professional development
- Total integrity

SCHOLARSHIPS

The Inns of Court, of which the Inner Temple is one, collectively award more than £5million annually in scholarships to students undertaking the Bar Professional Training Course (BPTC), which is the qualification required in order to practise as a barrister. The BPTC is undertaken after an undergraduate degree and takes a year to complete if it is studied full-time.

HOW TO GAIN RELEVANT WORK EXPERIENCE

Before committing yourself to a career at the Bar, it is wise to get an insight into what a barrister does. The best way to do this by undertaking work experience in the form of a 'mini pupillage' in a set of barristers' chambers. A mini pupillage usually lasts a week in which you might be reading papers, discussing cases, shadowing a barrister and attending court. Mini pupillages can help you to decide whether life as a barrister would suit you while also exposing you to areas of law you may wish to practise in at a later date. Relevant legal experience is also helpful, but undertaking at least three mini pupillages by the time you apply for pupillage is seen as a must. Pupillage refers to your first year of practise and is very competitive to secure. To apply for mini-pupillages, you can contact chambers directly or visit www.barcouncil.org.uk/careers/mini-pupillages/ which gives a directory of all the chambers in England and Wales. While you are in sixth form, you may also want to look into whether you are eligible to apply for the Bar Council's 'Bar Placement Week' and, during university, you should research the Inner Temple's Pegasus Access and Support Scheme. Both of these schemes offer students from underrepresented backgrounds the opportunity to undertake relevant work experience at the Bar.

For more in depth information, read the Inner Temple's 'Guide to becoming a Barrister', available on their website: www.innertemple.org.uk

MY EXPERIENCE

Baroness Helena Kennedy, QC, Doughty Street Chambers

"I grew up in Glasgow in a working class family, the first to go on to higher education. Neither of my older sisters had stayed on at school because family circumstances had made it impossible at the time. It was really through the encouragement of teachers that I decided to try for law and ended up coming to the Bar. I had no connections, no real understanding of how it all worked and found out it completely mystifying. However, I was unwilling to admit defeat and determined to succeed – even when I was told by sets of chambers that they did not take women – which they could do in those days!

At first I felt like a fish out of water because I had not gone to public school, was not male and I had an accent – which was very unusual then. However, I soon realised that my difference became my strength. My background gave me insight into the lives of many of the people for whom I acted and I had a ready empathy with the hard experiences of life that often brought people before the courts. In fact having an accent distinguished me from others and made me memorable, which was always a good thing at the Bar. They used to say ' Let's get that Scots girl' especially when Scotland supporters were arrested after cup finals having consumed too much alcohol or young Scotswomen had ended up on the game.

I have loved my life in the law. I think it is vital that people from hugely different backgrounds come into the profession because the law should have input from every quarter of our society. The knowledge that comes from diversity enriches law and make it more likely that law translated into justice. "

CAREERS IN IDEAS

www.careersinideas.org.uk

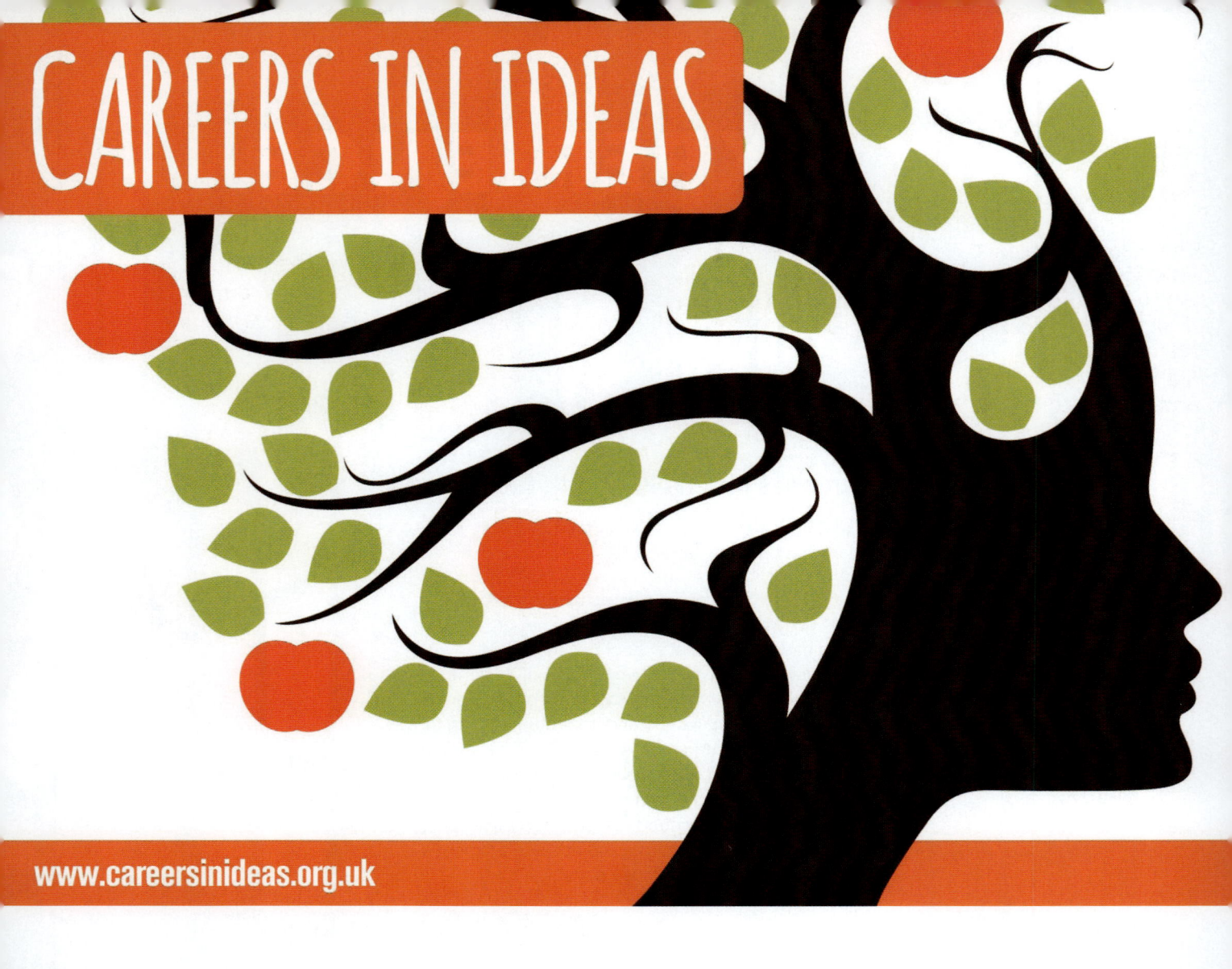

Careers in ideas

We all have ideas. And sometimes people will pay you for them. That's intellectual property. Intellectual Property, or 'IP', underpins so much of our society, from smartphones to the music on them, from textbooks to technology.

They all start with ideas.

Just like any other property, there are people who make a living buying and selling IP, helping others to make IP valuable, or finding ways to guard IP.

Some of these people are lawyers, some are business people or journalists. They work with inventors, scientists, artists and celebrities, as well as big technology companies and universities, to release the potential of ideas.

The pathways into the IP professions are as diverse as the jobs within the IP sector.

Qualifications in law, science, technology, engineering, maths or languages are helpful, and there are entry points into the IP sector for school-leavers and university graduates.

Visit www.careersinideas.org.uk to explore the diverse careers available in intellectual property.

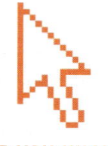

DID YOU KNOW?
Microsoft has a patent for opening a new window when you click a web link. It expires in 2021.

IP careers at a glance

There are many careers in ideas, including jobs suitable for school-leavers, 16-18 year olds, university graduates and postgraduates. Ownce you're in the IP profession, there are many opportunities for career progression.

Starting salaries for graduates usually exceed £25,000 and can rise to £100,000 or more within ten years.

The diagram below shows some of the careers in ideas and their entry points. In most cases, specific further training will be needed, which is often provided on the job.

There are thousands of jobs in the IP sector. Looking at one senior role alone, there are some 3,000 patent attorneys working in IP in all parts of the UK from London to Bristol, from Manchester to Aberdeen. Careers in ideas are also some of the most international careers, opening a world of opportunities.

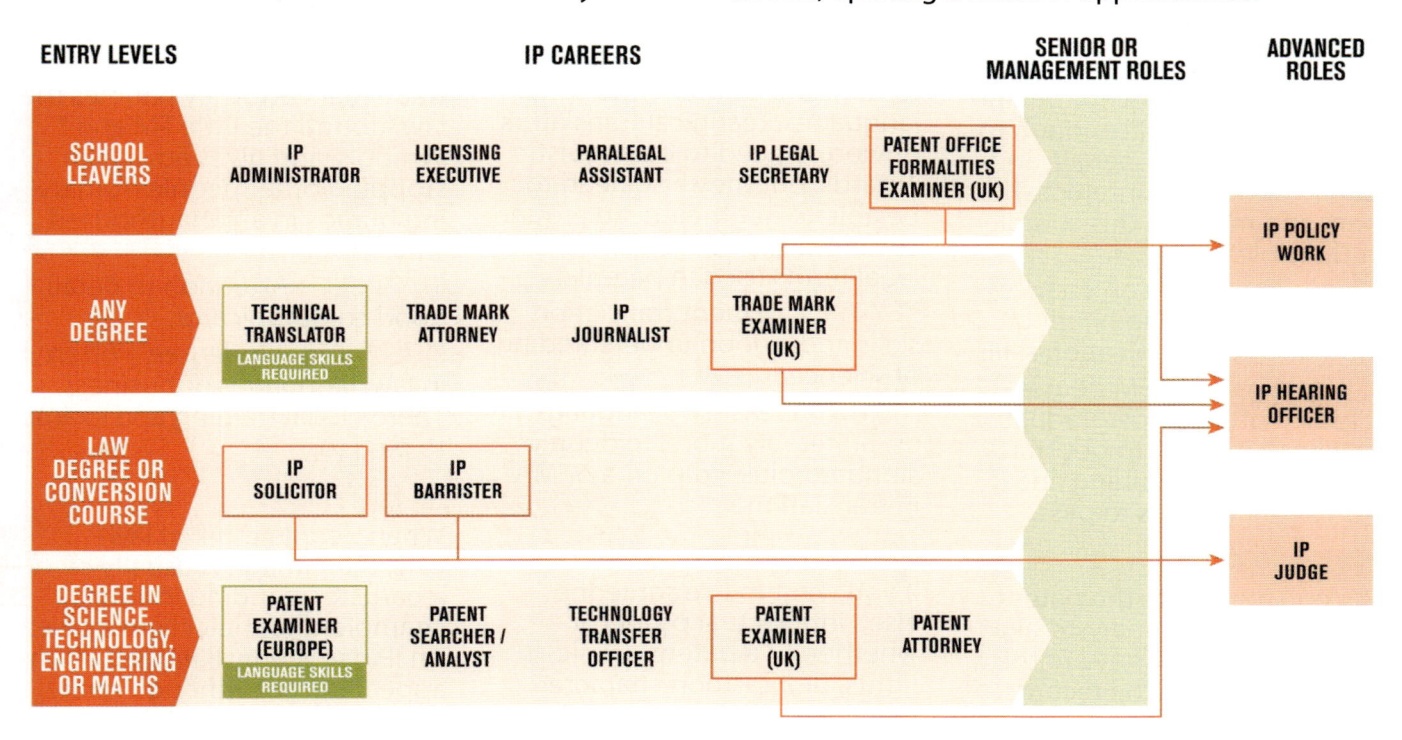

ENTRY LEVELS	IP CAREERS					SENIOR OR MANAGEMENT ROLES	ADVANCED ROLES
SCHOOL LEAVERS	IP ADMINISTRATOR	LICENSING EXECUTIVE	PARALEGAL ASSISTANT	IP LEGAL SECRETARY	PATENT OFFICE FORMALITIES EXAMINER (UK)		IP POLICY WORK
ANY DEGREE	TECHNICAL TRANSLATOR (LANGUAGE SKILLS REQUIRED)	TRADE MARK ATTORNEY	IP JOURNALIST		TRADE MARK EXAMINER (UK)		IP HEARING OFFICER
LAW DEGREE OR CONVERSION COURSE	IP SOLICITOR	IP BARRISTER					IP JUDGE
DEGREE IN SCIENCE, TECHNOLOGY, ENGINEERING OR MATHS	PATENT EXAMINER (EUROPE) (LANGUAGE SKILLS REQUIRED)	PATENT SEARCHER / ANALYST	TECHNOLOGY TRANSFER OFFICER	PATENT EXAMINER (UK)	PATENT ATTORNEY		

Jargon Buster

ATTORNEY Another word for a lawyer – someone with the appropriate legal qualifications to advise people on legal matters and represent them and their interests.

CHARTERED A 'chartered' professional – such as a chartered patent attorney – is someone who belongs to an organisation that protects the professionalism of their industry by keeping up standards of qualifications and client service. Being chartered is a sign that someone is properly qualified to provide advice (about patents, for instance), as they have to keep their skills and knowledge up-to-date to keep their chartered status.

INTELLECTUAL PROPERTY
Intellectual property – or 'IP' – is anything that might be worth something, but where the valuable bit is more of an idea than a physical object.
A house is 'property', because there's something physical there. The design for a house, on the other hand, is intellectual property because, even when it's drawn out on blueprints, it's the idea that's valuable, not the paper it's printed on.
Even once the house is built, intellectual property still exists in the design because that's what can be used to build more houses.

PARALEGAL A paralegal is a legal assistant – someone with a good enough understanding of the law to support the work of a qualified lawyer or attorney, but who's not qualified in law themselves.

R&D Short for 'research and development', this is about developing new product ideas, inventing, building prototypes, testing and refining. It's often top secret work at the cutting edge of technology. It can also be the name given to a department in a company which does this work.

STEM Short for 'science, technology, engineering and maths', STEM is often used to describe courses (at school or university) in any of these subjects similar to your own.

Graduate Careers

Patent attorney
Working in a law firm, in industry or in a government department, a patent attorney is a qualified legal practitioner who gets patents for clients, and helps them to realise their value and protect them. They have to be technical enough to understand the concept behind the inventions, legal enough to act on their clients' behalf, and human enough to interact with them and make all this complex stuff simple.
KEY SKILLS: Strong on science, mathematics or engineering and good communication skills.
NEEDS: A good STEM degree at least – often a postgraduate qualification too – to get started. There's legal training and professional exams to pass.

Patent analyst
Working alongside the patent attorneys are the analysts, aka patent searchers. They are the sleuths who hunt the records for similar ideas and inventions, checking for true originality. They're technical wizards, with data and engineering in their veins.
KEY SKILLS: Strong on science and maths, and a whizz at database search methods.
NEEDS: A good science degree.

Patent examiner
Like the patent analysts, the patent examiners check for originality, but the examiners work at the Patent Office, checking whether applications meet the standards to be awarded a patent. The UK Patent Office is in Newport in South Wales, but examiners are also needed at the European Patent Office's sites in Germany and the Netherlands.
KEY SKILLS: Super science insight, but also the power to explain.
NEEDS: A science, technology, engineering or maths degree with a high grade. (To work at the European Patent Office, some language skills are needed, although additional language training is available for new starters.)

Technical translator
Inventions can be complicated and technical, but patents for the inventions need to be easy to read and understand. When someone wants a patent in a non-English speaking country, a technical translator will need to translate a patent into other languages. Technical translators obviously need to be linguistic wizards, but they also need to be able to get their head around cutting-edge science and the legal terms used in patents.
KEY SKILLS: Fluent translation skills and a good understanding of science.
NEEDS: At least two languages, preferably more, to degree standard plus a diploma or MA in translation.

Licensing executive
If you want to use someone else's intellectual property – whether it's a patent, music rights, or a cartoon character that you want to put on a lunchbox – then you need to get a licence from them. Licensing executives are the wheeler dealers of the intellectual property world.
KEY SKILLS: A business and legal mind-set and excellent negotiation skills.
NEEDS: Usually you need a degree, preferably in law (or maybe in science for patent licensing), but depending on the IP area you're working in, there are many routes in.

Technology transfer officer
A lot of the best research goes on in universities. Sometimes research teams realise they've created something with a wider application. Technology transfer officers work with research teams – and often with outside companies – to commercialise academic ideas.
KEY SKILLS: A bit of science, a bit of law and a lot of business enterprise.
NEEDS: Typically a science degree, or a law or business degree together with a keen interest in science and technology.

Trade mark attorney
The trade mark attorney is the protector of brands – these include names and logos, and are used to distinguish between different goods or services. A trade mark attorney handles the law around the little TM and ® symbols, and gives advice on stopping other people from using brands in an unauthorised way.
KEY SKILLS: Attention to detail, good communicator.
NEEDS: A good degree – often in law, languages or business. There's legal training and exams to pass too.

IP barrister
When people think of lawyers, their image is usually of a barrister standing in court, championing their client's case. An IP barrister will indeed often appear in court (though rarely in front of a jury), arguing about IP issues that have reached a legal dispute. They also represent clients at other hearings and by providing advice about real or potential IP disputes.
KEY SKILLS: A persuasive communicator with a quick mind, willing to work hard.
NEEDS: A good degree in law or a different degree with a GDL (Graduate Diploma in Law). That qualifies you to start the Bar Professional Training Course and then start a 'pupillage' (on-the-job training). A-levels in science, or a degree in a STEM subject, can be a great background for a barrister who wants to specialise in patent cases.

IP solicitor
IP solicitors are where the legal mind meets the business brain. They advise and represent their clients in negotiations, disputes

and deals, doing everything from writing contracts to, sometimes, arguing cases in court.
KEY SKILLS: As well as the attention to detail of all lawyers, IP solicitors need the commercial understanding to see the big picture.
NEEDS: A good degree in law or a different degree with a GDL (Graduate Diploma in Law). That qualifies you to start the Legal Practice Course (LPC) and then start a two-year on-the-job training contract.

IP judge

After years of successful practice, some lawyers reach the top of the legal tree and sit as judges presiding over IP disputes and other legal cases. They might have to make decisions about patents, trade marks, design rights, copyright or all manner of associated legal issues, including who owns what rights and who's been infringing them.
KEY SKILLS: Knowledge, judgement and authority.
NEEDS: Many years of experience as a senior barrister or solicitor.

IP-related journalist

IP is a world of intrigues and innovations, breakthroughs and break-ups. Somebody needs to tell these stories, sometimes to the people who work in the sector, sometimes to the businesses, scientists and artists who need to understand it, and sometimes to the wider world.
KEY SKILLS: An inquiring mind, and a sharp writing style.
NEEDS: An understanding of the law and science could be helpful (but isn't a must). There are many routes to becoming a journalist, but it would be handy to have a degree and qualifications in law, science, business and/or journalism.

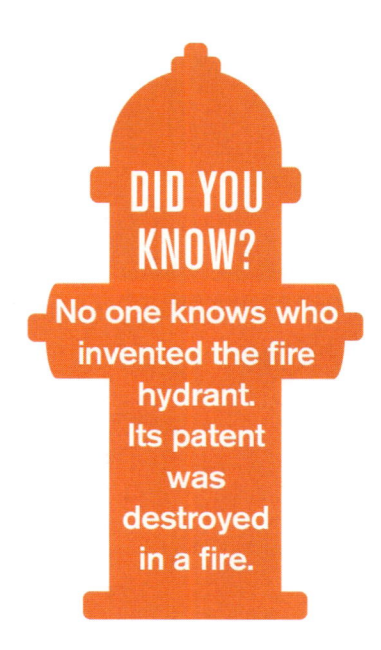

DID YOU KNOW? No one knows who invented the fire hydrant. Its patent was destroyed in a fire.

Ideas People

All sorts of people find fulfilling careers in IP, from different backgrounds in different roles. Meet some of those people here and hear their career stories from the world of ideas…

Chris Burnett, Patent Attorney

"I found out about the patent profession by chance whilst at university. Whilst I enjoyed my Biochemistry course, I preferred the theoretical and problem solving aspects to the practical side. I didn't want to work in a laboratory.

I have worked with multinational companies through to private inventors. The work can be very varied, with no two days the same. On one occasion I had to advise a manufacturer of cardboard Wendy houses on patent infringement. This entailed making Wendy houses in the office to compare them. On other occasions I get to advise pharmaceutical companies on legal aspects of their latest drugs. I work to ensure that our client's inventions are protected by securing patents and by enforcing patents once granted. It is fascinating to be involved from an invention's inception, where you must distil an idea into an underlying concept and cover all variations of the invention including future-proofing against new technologies that have not yet been invented."

Sarah Neil, Trade Mark Attorney

"I studied IP during my law degree and after deciding that the traditional solicitor/barrister route was not for me, but that I definitely wanted to work IP, I took to Google. A search for 'legal jobs in IP' introduced me to the concept of a Trade Mark Attorney, which had previously been completely unknown to both myself and my University careers advisor. I was able to meet a very kind Attorney willing to talk to me about the profession and helped me organise to gain some work experience.

I do a lot of work for well-known names in fashion and telecommunications. It's a great profession to allow you to build up a detailed knowledge of varied industries, some of which you might never have come across before. The job is also gives a real sense of accomplishment – nothing quite beats that feeling of walking down the high street, spotting a trade mark you have helped to register and thinking 'I was a part of making that happen.'"

ROCKETING TO THE MOON AND BEYOND

How current careers have now become the preparation for careers outside of the planet!

The future of careers is going beyond the boundaries of this very planet we live on. We shouldn't, however, be too hasty about life on the third rock from the sun, after all, before you can leap into space you would need to be able to handle the gravitational pull of earth!

So, that been said, we have some massive players in the space industry from National Aeronautics and Space Administration (NASA), European Space Agency (ESA), Russian Federal Space Agency and the China National Space Administration – all geared up for the next era of living and exploration. Over time institutions like NASA became so ingrained in popular culture the film and production industry has made references to them in award-winning productions. Space has not just been above and around us but entrenched in our lives. So, it is not unthinkable that the once unthinkable and unimaginable is now very much doable.

So much so that we have private companies and (wealthy) individuals embarking on space missions as the new trend and modern day (commercial) space race. Business adventurers like Bezos, Musk and Branson have taken their business arm wrestling to another level by funding missions that will take human beings to where probably only Neil Armstrong Yuri Gagarin had been decades ago.

Worth a read is A Galaxy of Her Own by Libby Jackson who is current the Human Spaceflight & Microgravity Programme Manager at the UK Space Agency.

Examples of such planned trips to outer space range from:

Mars One
mars-one.com

Hyperloop One
hyperloop-one.com

Virgin Galactic
virgingalactic.com

European Space Agency
ESA.int

National Aeronautics and Space Administration
NASA.com

Blue Origin
blueorigin.com

SpaceX
spacex.com

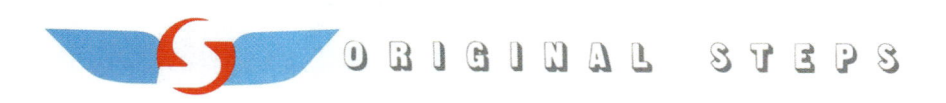

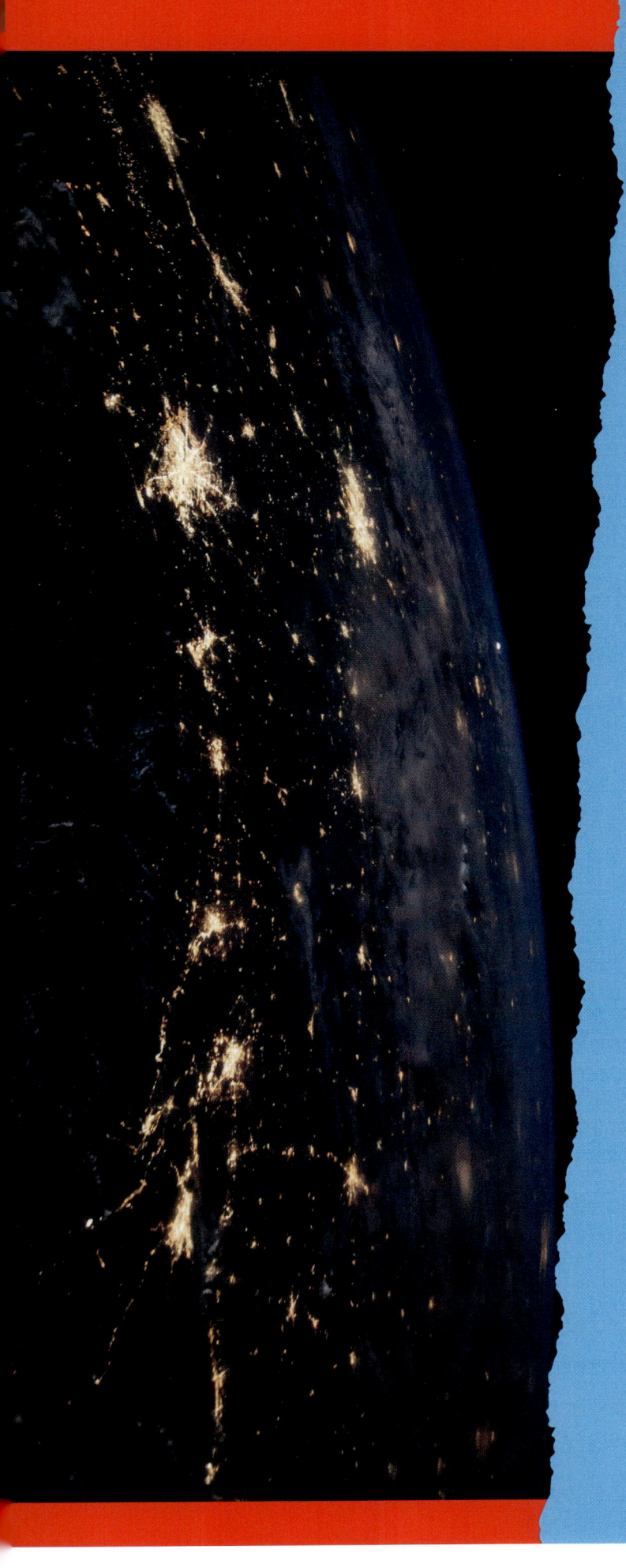

If you are wealthy enough to splash out for the trip, your best bet would be to pursue a career in the industry. Though a career as an astronaut would be awesome, not many are able to pursue this path. The few who do, enter into this field from the get go - either directly entering through programs within various national platforms like NASA or join the air force to become a pilot with the idea of changing equipment from that of the defence force to that of a space program. Others (especially with a fear of heights) can tackle the engineering field in Aeronautics and pursue their ambitions within this sector – while staying grounded.

The NASA astronaut program is known to be intense but but provides the foundation to prepare for a potentially challenging task as being an intergalactic traveller. Afterall, if it was that easy, everyone would do it!

Find out more:
astronauts.nasa.gov

Again, to emphasise, not everyone is able to qualify or be employed by NASA, ESA etc. So instead of being status quo about it, one can be rather proactive and prepare for the potential careers to arise once space travel becomes an everyday activity...

ORIGINAL STEPS

Let's look at the present and then guesstimate the future of careers...in space!

Hospitality

Waiters, bar staff, hotel managers, airline staff, chefs and their crew. These are all very much the cornerstone career paths of the hospitality industry. These jobs rely heavily on tourism and travel! This extends to business, recreational and cultural events – the industry is a booming heartbeat in earth's financial cross currency exchange.

Individuals can study for years at various culinary schools, doing apprenticeships on cruise-liners and even doing the clean-up duties on the night shift at various events to make ends meet and clock valuable experience hours. Learning how to deal with customers, address happenings at events and being able to manage entire hotels. The hospitality industry is an ecosystem that stretches from land to sea and air and soon space!

Several universities and colleges specialise in the hospitality industry by offering degree-based programs. These programs the like of The Blue Mountains International Hotel Management School in Australia has served up some of the world's best talent in this sector. The International Hotel School from South Africa for instance, has further taken the leap by pushing hospitality education through the continent of Africa. These institutions are providing launch pads to the next level of tourism. So perhaps soon a course or two or how to serve a drink in zero gravity could be added to the curriculum!

Airlines

On the ground, companies like Easy Jet are cleverly generating a keen interest in the future, by taking small steps (as Armstrong once put it) and building electric powered aircraft for commercial passenger jet travel.

So, if you are looking at becoming a pilot now - start by checking out options at various flight schools to complete your PPL (Private Pilot's Licence) as your step up to pursuing your (CPL) Commercial Pilots Licence. Another good example is the highly competitive entry point of airline pilot academies. Though difficult to get into, it is a world-class option of having your training paid for you.

Check out:

The British Airways Cadet Programme - jobs.ba.com/jobs/futurepilot/

Another option is to consider a national air force training program such as the Royal Airforce - www.raf.mod.uk/

With the amount of airlines merging, being acquired or being closed, the industry has become mired with a haphazard wave of uncertainty for a very demanding sector! So, what will future careers in the airline industry look like?

As current ground staff and flight controllers, keep airports in check and make sure travel is timely managed, the future will have people managing travel remotely in mission control centres or in floating or orbiting stations.

The creative industry

A while back NASA put together a campaign called the Visions of the Future and provided an almost retro visionary feel to the future of modern living beyond earth. Lands of opportunities and new beginnings, advertised to the everyday person yearning for a better life.

To have a glimpse, visit:

www.jpl.nasa.gov/visions-of-the-future

It is also a campaign that was driven and cultivated by the creative industry capturing aspects of the very unknown. How the marketing, design and creative industry sets the pace for the pending new world ahead is something not to be overlooked. As the advertising industry moves and shapes itself into mediums such as new media and digital outlays, what lies in the future for the creative minds? Perhaps campaigns and adverts branded on the moon?, Perhaps the new method of advertising will go beyond traditional mediums which in our present day is TV, Internet and mobile. The exciting part is that one can really go ballistic as the universe provides a canvas for countless ideas beyond our imagination. We will be looking no further than the creative thinkers from the comic book industry, who, for years they have been advocating for life and adventures in realms unknown to us all. Furthermore, films like Star Wars and Star Trek already provided the concept of modern man living in space and not far-fetched as we are already using some of the things we marvelled about in Back to the Future and the space age movies.

Geologists vs Quantity Surveyors

Finally after years of digging around the rock we call earth, people of the planet are now finally becoming experts in rock-´et´ science (excuse the pun). For years, man has been digging holes on the planet, but now the universe is now providing new forms of rocks and minerals that may provide better renewable alternatives beyond fossil fuels. Quantity Surveyors are needed to count bricks, not quite literally speaking but still their skills are very useful, and between them and geologists, they have a lot of work ahead of them to help build and create new ways of living and thriving on other planets.

Architects

One doesn't have to look further than the architectural designs and creations of the late Zaha Hadid and Tom Wright to see the world is ready to transport home-grown masterpieces to showcase on other home planets.

The world is ready to go beyond itself, yes infrastructure and development on earth is still very much reliant on the advent of changing ecosystem and weather patterns and physical changes to the earths crust. And we still have a lot to do to make sure the earth survives, as it seems at times the inhabitants of the world are its very own worst enemies. But the future looks awesome and the life beyond our current terra-firma may be, perhaps for the ones reading this now, be out of reach but passing on what we know now and what we are developing via our interesting careers to our future generations is critical to setting up the advent of living amongst the stars!

So be inspired - look at careers differently, see the world full of opportunities and options, and think bigger. Discover the route to those possibilities, whether it be a doctor, engineer or a teacher (the world always needs teachers and good teachers too - Oprah said so and she used to giving things away for free on television so it is true!), whatever your career aspirations are, do the research find what study option is best suited for you and go make it happen - but with a broader (out of this world) outlook.

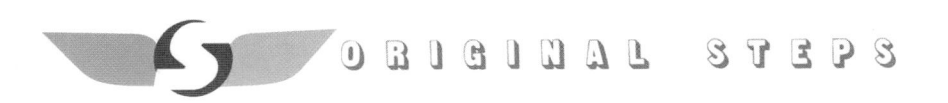

RUN YOUR BUSINESS LIKE A MOVIE

Stepping up to be the lead character of your own adventure

Watching a blockbuster film that has all the adrenaline and emotional inducing effects and more than often meets the expectations of viewers who pay good money to be seated with popcorn and a favourite beverage, for an exciting escape from reality for several minutes. And even after the film, for a few minutes, one tends to romanticise about the heroes they have seen and draft real-life adventures based on these fictional personas. From heartbreak to success, a film often sets the tone for a micro-version of what can happen when starting up a business from scratch!

And just like a well-scripted feature, starting a business can be depicted as the quest by the "underdog" or "champion on the rise" in a movie looking to achieve what most couldn't.

The perception that creating a business is difficult and that pursuing a career in a more structured environment is no doubt the more popular route for many. After all, many of the companies that individuals go to seek employment at, were started off in very similar styles and ended up growing into job-creating empires.

Our focus, however, is on the next generation - the new adventurers seeking to springboard new empires and create employment for others. And the questions that need to be addressed for them would be: How, Why, Where and What.

Going into business:

Well just like in a film, there first needs to be a reason to embark on an adventure. Unlike an action adventure which is usually sparked up by love or the ever-popular quest for revenge, a business (hopefully) is prompted when an individual or group of individuals see a gap in the market to address and grow an enterprise in the process.

Now a gap in the market could be a need for a product or even a need to be a competitor to stimulate a market and the scripting of a screenplay resembles the development of a business plan.

The business plan, however, unlike the screenplay

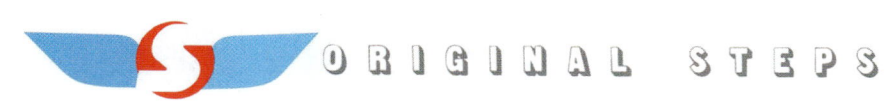

generally doesn't always go according to plan. It does create an understanding of where and what the business will be doing and the direction in which it will take to achieve it and usually is created to attract funders and shareholders.

The next concern would be how one can create a business out of a plan and that largely relies on capital to build a product, an app or service providing mechanism in the first place. Individuals can start with a small amount of capital and resources and then while they grow, reinvest into the business, while others depending on the scope of the offering will need larger amounts. This seed (starting) capital can be broken down into the following:

1. Savings (your own capital)

2. Microloans from family and friends.

3. Bank loans (this will need a form of security to secure the financing)

4. Social media - the popular crowdfunding route

5. Individual or private investors - individuals who gain shareholding in a business for a capital injection.

6. Government grants and funding schemes.

7. Angel investors, accelerator funds, incubators and venture capital funds - this is often benched against an equity

By investing that capital back into the business one can drive a business forward and is a key determinant of the sustainability of the business – something that is often overlooked to the detriment of many start-ups.

But just like the adventures on the big screen, it is never a smooth ride and the hero does make mistakes, takes further risks and sometimes never recovers. The next twist, chapter or sequel tends to either make or break the individual, dusting oneself off and being able to head into the next challenge is critical.

Whatever the case may be, starting a business will never provide a dull day. The opportunities and paths that one can drive ranges from job creations, market stimulations, generating capital and of course a successful career path.

The key is - just like a well-directed production needs an outstanding and award-winning lead character, so does a business. Are you ready to take the lead?

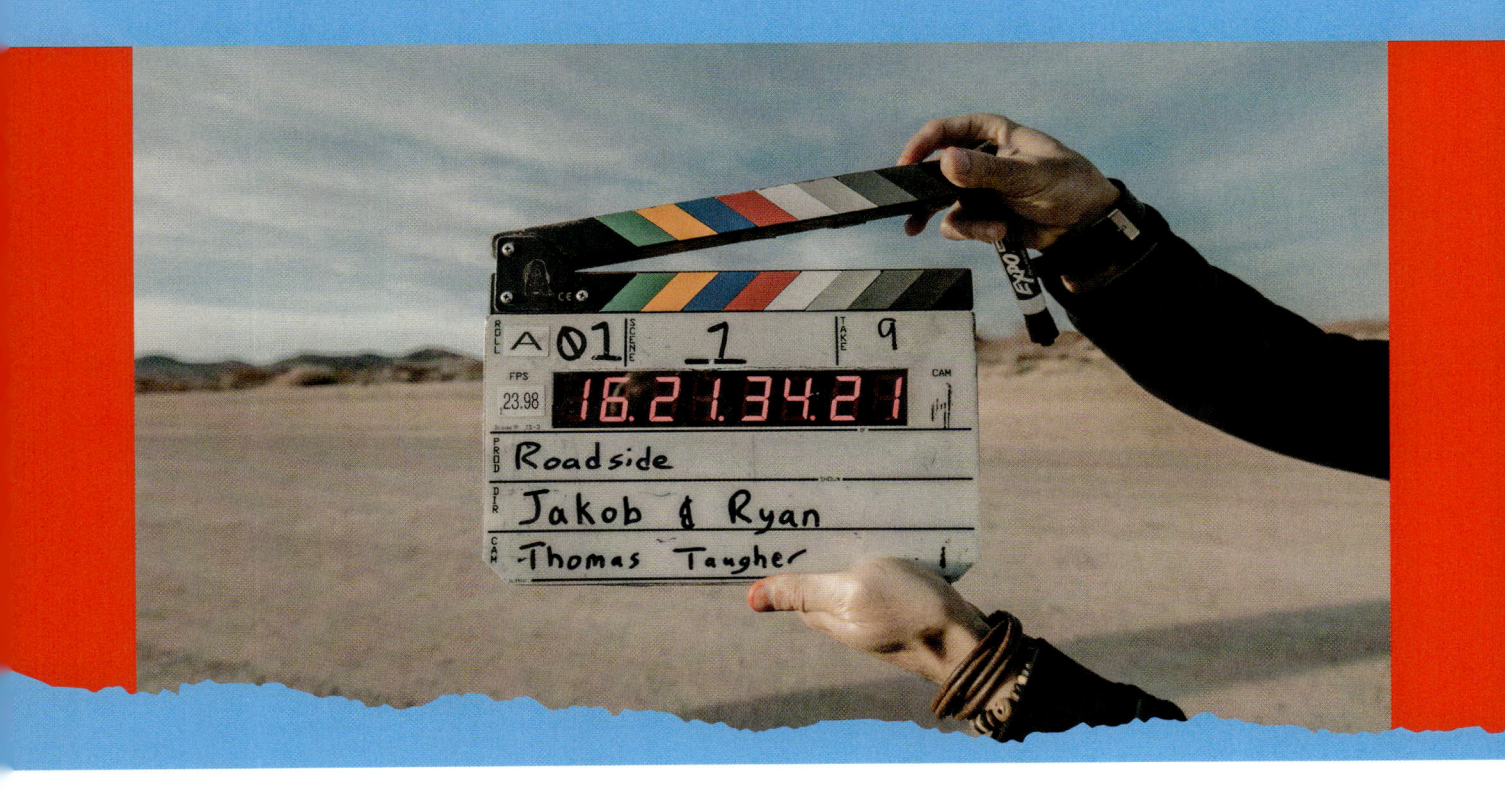

ORIGINAL STEPS

GAME OF CAREERS

Trying to make sense of the game of career (hunting) - the playing field has been levelled...

Globally the world has become a lot smaller, and not from a crazy shrinking ray from a planet full of evil aliens looking to take over the earth. Okay, so we have been watching way too many superhero films!

Getting back to the point we were trying to make, the world, and in a more lucid description, has become more interconnected. Technology has brought about such a powerful channel for diversification of human capital skills and job requirements that the old methods in the past that worked so well for so many, just doesn't quite cut the mustard anymore.

So as the world trends move rapidly and dynamically, individuals, both young and old, battle to keep up on the job scene.

There is no more a fine blueprint or fairy tale step-by-step guide - just real life throwing challenges at individuals who not only have to keep up with the responsibilities of a career but also manage everything else revolving around it. From the first world to the third world, young and old, single to married, healthy to disabled, the list of situations and statuses is plentiful...one thing remains the pursuit of a career. And yes, there the odd or unfortunate ones that make a career of being unemployed!

The playing field has certainly been levelled and competition is much bigger...

According to the International Labour Organization (ILO) in 2016, it was estimated 199,4 million people where globally unemployed and that in 2017 it would jump up a further 1,1 million.

Whilst the according to the Yale University publication, YaleGlobal Online, the world is in literally spinning into a financial earthquake based on the student loan debt.

The USA alone has racked up an estimated student debt figure that has flown over the Trillion Dollar mark.

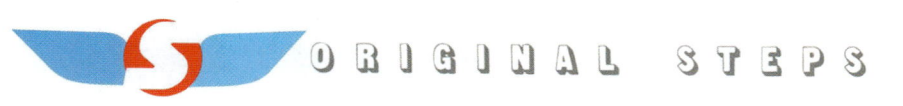

And with the world being ever so connected the job market that was once localized has become a staging ground for companies to draft talent from various parts of the planet to serve their needs within their requirements.

Okay so let's recap – we have gone from a small planet, mentioned aliens with shrink rays, superheroes, global unemployment, a student debt crisis, fast-moving technology (FMT), mustard and a trillion odd dollars!

Confused, shocked, scared? I mean, how is someone supposed to choose a career that effectively has a massive impact on his or her life given the above-mentioned obstacles? It isn't as easy as it used to be, and sure, the traditional LAD system (Lawyer, Accountant, and Doctor), provided a stable career base and that individuals could strive to attain, but it was not always accessible to many. In addition, though rewarding, not everyone is able to be a lawyer, accountant or doctor, and let's not forget engineers. Structural engineers are supposed to make things stable so stability is quite literally part of their career spec. Quantity surveyors count bricks and geologists specialize in hard stones. Poor stereotypes aside, these stable careers aren't as attractive as they once seemed, nor as financially rewarding.

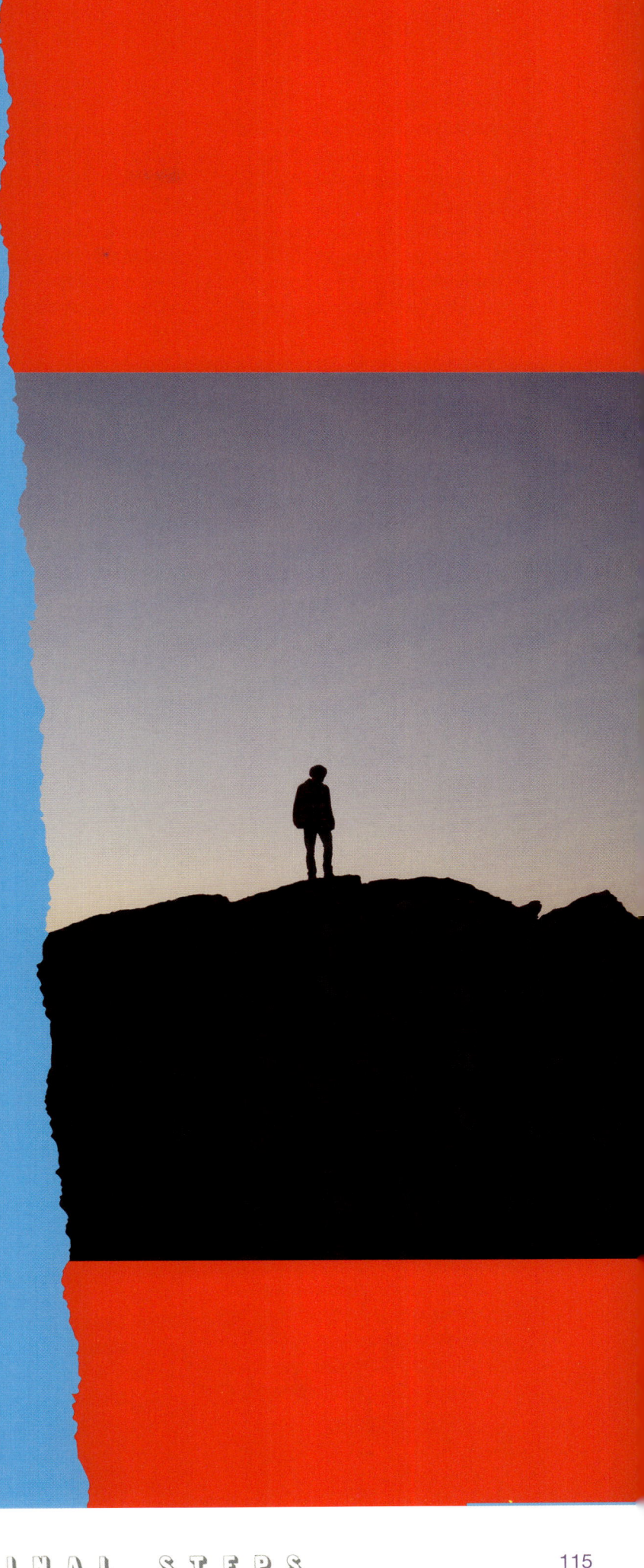

Thanks to the advancement of modern technology and Artificial Intelligence (AI) world needs more creative individuals, inventors of future technologies, solvers of problems and public leaders. The world as small as it seems and as fast as it is spinning – needs individuals from all sectors and not just the ones from the LAD system.

So, let's break it down:

What is the backbone of a career?

Education, this is the key factor in any career. From a basic education qualification to a fundamental higher education of pure academics. The world has systemically created levels of skills. And just like in a game the more levels you pass the more skilled you become in the ability to clock the game!

Choosing the right education path, however, opens a whole other equation. Reading for a qualification in law, for instance, is often perceived as a defining point for a career. Or is it? Does a person who studies law have to practice law? Does the actual educational institution have an impact on a career? The answer solely lies within the individual and what their objectives are.

Naturally, an individual educated at an Ivy league university is typically exposed to more opportunities than others through a robust alumni network and close-knit connections, however, the concept of leading a horse to water seemingly applies.

In most cases, however, for other individuals, getting a career or job is driven by financial or personal responsibilities – which are often so heavy, that the option of the perfect career choice is out of reach (but not impossible!).

Putting it into the practice – the playing field becomes well and truly open...

The world of careers is an unprotected environment, a far drift away from the safety of the classroom, lecturer room, and study hall. Individuals need to compete and to be able to survive or succeed in a highly pressurized environment.

Also, before you think you are throwing your books away for good once you enter the job market, the learning never stops. You will need to constantly hone your skills and objectives to stay relevant in a dynamic jobs environment.

So, if an educational path and choosing an actual career is to be determined by and chosen by in the long run by you, how should individuals decide what is best for themselves?

Research, ask and do: build your own database of information

The great part of this technology-driven world we live in, is that the Internet is quite literally at our fingertips – so vast is the nature of the technology there is even a union assigned to it! International Telecommunication Union (ITU - itu.in). Google has become a go-to research hub, for the first point of contact to information platforms. So, get researching and explore the options available online to save you the time and effort going out (to libraries and job centres) to do so. Check out various industries and companies, understand what employers look for and learn from successful individuals. Read, watch and listen your way forward.

According to Investopedia, the top ten highest paid jobs in the world ranges from being a surgeon to being a pharmacist.

If you still can't find the right answer then speak to a relevant career counsellor or professional in a field of your interest and ask as many questions as you can.
Next up: experience the field – internships, work practicals, volunteering - get a feel for what you are looking to get into before you take the leap!

Be inspired: Watch films and documentaries or read up about leaders in various fields of your interest to get an understand what it takes to work in an industry – and though the films need to be taken with a few pinches of salt naturally, they do a good job at getting you fired up for that position of your dreams.

The trending talent pools:

Graduate Recruitment Programmes

have become the career bridging system of fresh talent from higher education into corporates. The marketing and impact of these programs have become a big factor for graduates looking to gain employment upon qualifying.

Start-ups

the business path for young individuals with little to risk and everything to gain has become an attractive idea of making it big quick and making it rich fast but in a sustainable way....

The career sidestep

the individual who decides to do something different after journeying down a specific avenue.

The key, is to make an informed and well-researched decision, just like in a game of speed chess where every move counts though the clock is ticking! Thinking before acting is the best way to outwit or outsmart in the career game!

Example of newer careers:

Hospitality

A career in Beer – become a brewer or start your own microbrewery!

Travel and Logistics

A career in space – become an astronaut! NASA or the ESA provides a starting point for research.

Environment

Stop poaching and help save the planet – become a geneticist! Check out the ICUN Red List - iucnredlist.org

Communications

Social media has made that a truly open field – however, good journalism is what helps keeps the planet informed. Read up about Bob Woodward and Carl Bernstein as game-changing examples.

Entertainment and Sport

Quite simply show me the money! - watch Jerry McGuire or Money Ball and get a glimpse of how intense this sector is.

Launched in 2005 OriginalSteps.com is a leading online resource providing information on Careers, Education, Startups, Student Finance and Gap Years. Powered by the producers of the Breaking Stereotypes documentary project and the Fun Side of Being Serious book series.

Visit: www.OriginalSteps.com or connect via contact@OriginalSteps.com

The JobCrowd

WHY REGISTER?

We create the only ranking of graduate and apprentice employers based on employees feedback. Early career candidates use our media platforms to research TOP COMPANIES they want to work for....

How?

97% of early career candidates are more likely to apply to top companies

Over 2 million annual visitors to www.theJobCrowd.com

APPLY

THE JOB APPLICATIONS SECTION

APPLY

2018

WORK EXPERIENCE

Work experience is an important way to work out what you might like to do as a future career, develop skills which will be of use in any working environment and potentially supplement your income whilst you are studying. In today's competitive job market, it's a necessity to have work experience on your CV, but finding relevant work experience (either paid or unpaid) is not an easy task. And just how 'relevant' does it need to be? Read about some of the different types of work experience, and how to get your foot in the door.

INSIGHT EVENTS OR WEBINARS

Although not strictly work experience, these are fantastic opportunities to get involved in. The selection criteria is generally less strict than for formal programmes, so you have a higher chance of getting in – you just have to ensure you're on the right mailing lists so that you get notified of them when they launch. You can sign up for alerts about these sort of events on the Pure Potential website (www.purepotential.org). They are usually short and snappy – designed to give you an idea of what the career entails and the kind of candidates they are looking for, and to entice you to apply!

VOLUNTEERING

Doing voluntary work with a registered charity or non-governmental organisation shows passion and integrity, as well as motivation because you will be doing it without being paid, although your expenses will be reimbursed. The experience will be rewarding, and will provide you with an opportunity to develop skills that are important to future employers too. Charities are always looking for people to help out, so this kind of experience is easier to get than others.

WORK SHADOWING

Observing someone in their role can be an effective way to decide whether a certain career is really for you, in just a few days. You will gain experience of real, high level work and be able to talk about a role and industry with someone on the job. Shadowing is a more informal type of work experience, and tends to be the norm in creative industries where there is a looser and smaller structure to the business, such as film and television production, publishing, journalism or marketing. The downside to this type of placement is that it can be unstructured, so could involve a lot of administrative work without much 'real' experience. However, even if you don't get that much responsibility, these placements can be great in terms of the contacts you make and people you meet and getting an idea of what the job entails.

INTERNSHIPS

This kind of work experience is structured and paid, though often involves a highly competitive application process. Internships consist of a fixed period of work within a company, during which you may be given quite a high degree of personal responsibility. Investment banks, for example, tend to run programmes in the spring and summer holidays, and the bigger law firms have an equivalent programme called a 'vacation scheme'. Application deadlines tend to be several months in advance, so don't leave things too late. They will also want to see evidence of other work experience.

HOW TO...SUCCESSFULLY SECURE WORK EXPERIENCE

DO THE RESEARCH

Identify the industry in which you wish to sample through work experience; be sure that any company you write to offers the role that appeals to you and is a place you'd like to work.

BE SPECIFIC

Always try to address your letters to a person rather than a 'Dear Sir/Madam'. You are much more likely to get a response.

CALL

Telephone the organisation and ask if they need any temporary help. Send a CV with a covering letter or covering email.

ASK AROUND

What do your parents, friends' parents, teachers, tutors do? Can they help or put you in touch with someone? State your availability. Give a potential start date and indicate how long you can work for.

PERSEVERE

You might not succeed at finding a volunteering opportunity straight away, but don't be put off. Keep persevering to find a placement that suits you and that is in a field you are interested in.

BE WILLING

Offer to volunteer, even for just a few hours. If that doesn't work ask if you can buy them a coffee, or even just have a 15 minute phone conversation – who knows what doors this might open...

GAP YEAR PROGRAMMES

Some firms offer programmes where you can work in your gap year, enabling you to earn some money, acquire new skills and get a taste of the working world over a prolonged period before you start university. These programmes are not only an excellent addition to your personal statement, but also will stand you in good stead when it comes to finding a job once you have graduated if you decide to go to university. Participating in one of these programmes will show you have ambition, are motivated and take your career seriously, and who knows - if you excel during the programme the firm may offer you a job nobody forgets a keen and enthusiastic employee!

HOW RELEVANT DOES IT NEED TO BE?

Many students worry about finding work experience which is relevant to their university course or future career, however, we all know that finding these opportunities can be difficult, and that you might change your mind later down the line – does that mean the work experience you've done is irrelevant? NO! Finding any type of work experience which builds upon your key skills is far better than nothing at all. It's about the skills you develop whilst on your work experience that counts more than the companies you did work experience at.

MAKE CONTACTS

After any work experience you do, make sure you take down the contact details of all the people you met – you never know when these might come in handy, or when your paths may cross again. During the placement be a pleasure to work with and always go the extra mile by being proactive, staying that little bit later, offering your assistance to everyone you meet, and be somebody they would want to see again in the future. At the end, thank them for giving you the opportunity, and if anyone has been particularly kind or useful then a box of chocolates or bunch of flowers will ensure they remember you.

EMPLOYABILITY SKILLS

Meesh Nah
Course Manager – *filtered.com*

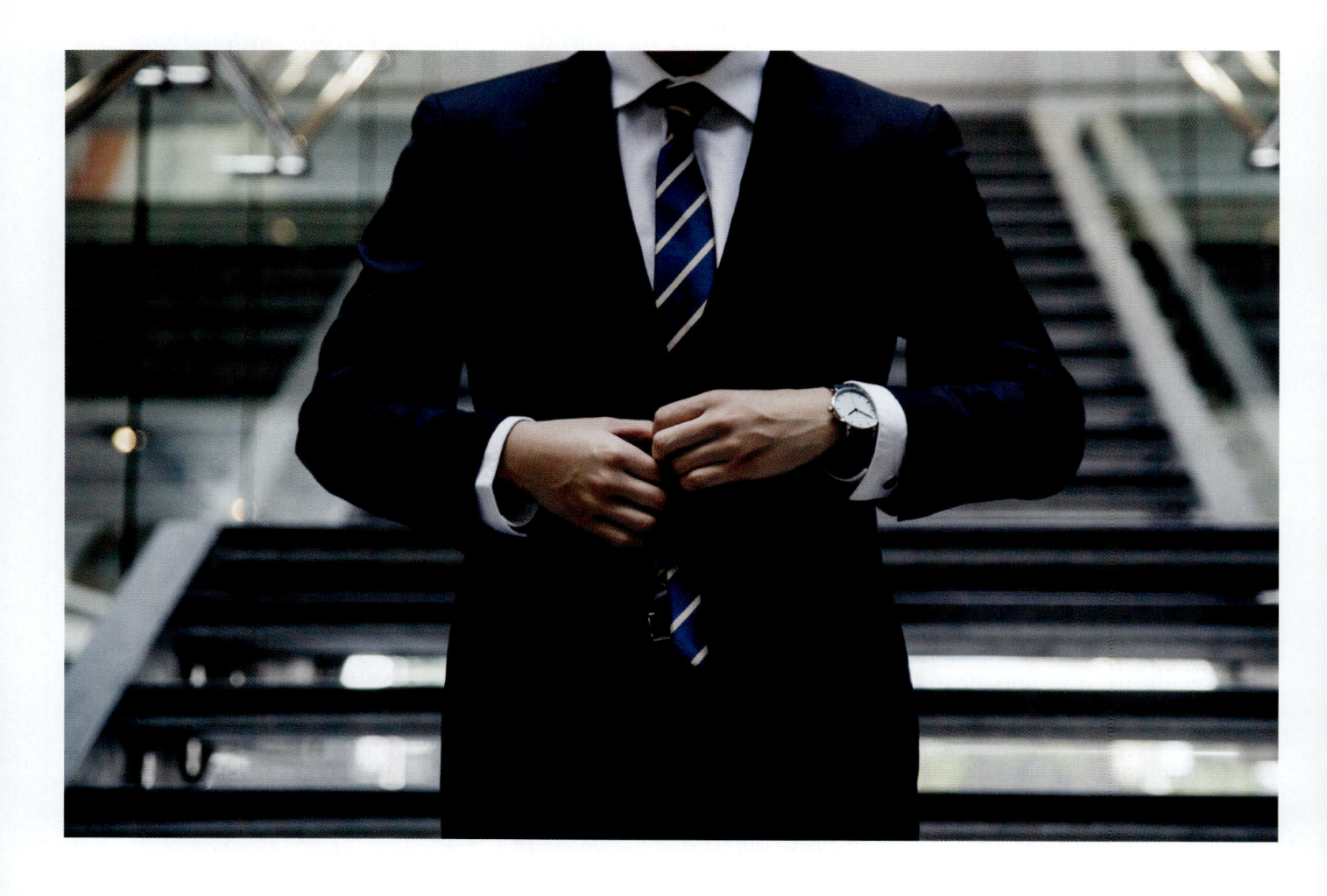

Employability skills are also known as transferable skills. Why are they important? Formal qualifications paint a picture of your abilities, but employability skills demonstrate the quality of you as a potential employee.

Whilst there is a defined finishing line to formal qualifications (i.e. when you pass and get a grade!), with employability skills there is very rarely a limit; you can always learn and develop more.

That is not to say there aren't courses in these skills. There are, and you can also attain professional qualifications. But it important to remember that you can show evidence for having these skills with the jobs and experiences that you have had in the past. You can improve these skills on an ongoing basis.

Let's take a look these skills.

COMMUNICATION VERBAL & WRITTEN

Communication is both the ability to take in information (listening) and the ability to give out information (verbally or in writing). It is an essential part of building relationships and achieving goals along with others. Demonstrating the ability to listen and carry out instructions, as well as being able to assess the appropriate way to communicate in a business environment is one of the most important qualities that employers look for in their workers.

TEAMWORK

A good team works with the strengths and weaknesses with each individual member. Being able to work effectively and harmoniously with a diverse group of people to achieve shared goals is key to success in any business. So employers look for people who can contribute positively to the team they will be joining by supporting others when needed and being understanding of differences when faced with challenges.

COMMERCIAL AWARENESS

Commercial awareness is about having an understanding about the industry / sector that a company works within, as well as knowledge about any relevant subjects. This could be new technologies, laws, competitors, the current economy, who the customers are – the list is long, as companies don't exist in isolation so it's important to see how their relationships to other factors influence the decisions that are made. Having commercial awareness will also help you to understand why you are doing the work you are being asked to do so

ANALYSING & RESEARCH

Being able to analyse and research means both being able to look for materials and being able to take in materials that are given to you (this could be in the form of an article to a large spreadsheet of data) to read and find key information within them. Analysing also means being able to assess what you are digesting and being able to see gaps or form opinions about what you are reading or seeing or hearing.

CREATIVE THINKING & PROBLEM SOLVING

Coming up with solutions often requires both logical and creative thinking. A challenge can often be resolved by analysing relevant information or data, followed by using your creative thinking skills to come up with practical ideas to figure out how to avoid the same issue reoccurring. It's important to be able to do this as part of a team, so taking into consideration the needs of others, as well as the needs of the business (commercial awareness).

SELF-MOTIVATION

Also known as drive and taking initiative. When you are self-motivated, you work without being pressured or influenced by other people or external situations (such as deadlines!). You want the responsibility of wanting to do well for yourself and for your team. This could be demonstrated by starting or finishing a task or project even when it can be difficult, or by being proactive about the skills you need to get or improve on to progress in your life.

PLANNING & ORGANISING

Also known as time management. Being able to plan and organize your tasks around the time that you have is a really important skill. It demonstrates an element of self-motivation too. Being practical and realistic in being able to see what steps you need to take in order to complete a task and how long each step will take (and sticking to it where possible and being honest when you can't!) will ensure your employer gains trust in your abilities.

THE PURE POTENTIAL CV WRITING MASTERCLASS

`Curriculum Vitae means 'the course of one's life' in Latin and is one of several methods used by employers to select candidates.`

We like to think of a CV as a personal marketing document – it offers employers a snapshot of who you are and sells your strengths, achievements and any relevant work experience you've gained. It doesn't matter how amazing you are or how much of an asset you would be to a company, if you can't communicate it through your CV, you certainly won't get very far. This is exactly why you must spend time creating a high-quality CV, which you regularly update.

The majority of employers will ask for a CV, along with a supporting covering letter which clearly outlines exactly why you are applying for a particular role, why you want to work for that firm and what makes you the perfect candidate. There's plenty of advice on writing a covering letter later on, but let's focus on the CV to begin with

WHAT GOES IN YOUR CV?

A concise CV is extremely important when it comes to making a positive first impression – no recruiter wants to read pages and pages of information. Never let your CV expand beyond two sides of A4, preferably one side (yes, we are being serious). In fact, even the CV's of middle-aged professionals with a lot more experience under their belts than trainees are often kept to just one side of A4. Your CV should include only the most important bits of relevant information about you that relate to the job in question – check out the CV template for a breakdown of the core sections.

There are many good ways of structuring a CV, and this will vary depending on how much experience you have and what stage of your career you're at. The rules are to be clear, concise but comprehensive.

SECTION ONE: THE BASICS

Include your name, address, contact number and email. Don't include a photo or your date of birth, and there is no need to provide a middle name unless you use it. Make sure your email address sounds professional; 'funkyfairy@' or 'gangsta_lolz@' is not going to impress. Your name should be the title, not 'CV'.

SECTION TWO: SUMMARISE WHO YOU ARE

Some people like to have a 2-4 sentence summary that outlines their key skills and attributes, but some prefer not to. Either way it is a good exercise to get you thinking about what you have to offer and what makes you unique.

EXERCISE: Ask a good friend or family member to think of up to five words to describe you. We're talking positive words here! We are not looking for things like 'hilarious' or a 'good sport', but more along the lines of the following:
Hard-working, Reliable, Patient, Trustworthy, Committed, Determined, Meticulous, Well-presented, Professional, Effective communicator, Efficient, Adaptable, Independent, Confident, Mature

Once you've finalised a few words you feel truly represent you then turn this into sentences, and add what you hope to do. For example:

"I am a hard-working, determined person with a professional attitude. My ability to communicate effectively makes me an asset to any team. I am looking for a role within the retail sector to gain valuable work experience."

SECTION THREE: EDUCATION

The employer only wants to see your secondary education, so no nursery or primary school information please! Enter your education in reverse chronological order, so put what you're doing now first, and work your way backwards. Always include the date, and if you're still studying put the date e.g. '2014 – present'. If you are currently taking A-Levels or equivalent then list each subject and the grade achieved. If you haven't got any grades yet then you may wish to enter your predicted grades, followed by '(predicted)', but this is not compulsory.

Unless they have specified any particular subjects for GCSE (sometimes they want to know your Maths and English grade) you don't need to tell them all your subjects, just a summary such as '5As, 3Bs and 1C' should suffice. If you have taken any other qualifications which would count under education then enter them here too.

SECTION FOUR: WORK EXPERIENCE

Again, list your work experience in reverse chronological order. It can be hard to decide what to put down here. Much of the work experience you have done already may not be at all relevant to the job you are applying to, but that's absolutely fine. As a sixth former you are not expected to have done industry-specific work, but what you do want to show is that you are willing to work hard. Have confidence in the character building work you've done and don't dismiss valuable work experience because you don't think it will make you stand out. Employers value young people who are willing to do unglamorous work – it shows you have tenacity, commitment and drive, and are willing to start at the bottom. Start by including everything you've ever done! You can always edit things out later.

Many young people complete work experience immediately after their GCSEs, this can be a good place to start. If you've helped a family member in some way then you can include that too, any menial work or manual labour could count, so jot down everything you've done, from paper boy/girl, assisting at a baker or butcher, stacking shelves, mowing lawns, dog-walking and baby-sitting to making tea and photocopying in an office - it could all count! Don't go too far back though, it should not include anything before Year 10 unless it is particularly relevant.

EXERCISE: Once you have listed the work experiences you have done you need to make whatever you did sound as professional and worthwhile as possible by using what we call 'Power Verbs'. These tell the recruiter what you are doing, or did - make sure you get the tense right! It can feel odd to use these words to describe something you consider easy but it shows the prospective employer that you recognise the skills you have picked up – a sure sign of maturity. Here are some examples to get you started:

Organising, Consulting, Negotiating, Presenting, Managing, Booking, Attending, Writing, Working, Liaising, Assisting, Creating, Producing, Helping, Ensuring, Participating, Communicating, Shadowing, Transferring, Analysing, Reading, Overseeing

SECTION FIVE: PERSONAL DEVELOPMENT

Anything that isn't employment, but is helping you to develop as a young adult should go in this section. Mention any voluntary work you do, awards you have won, or positions of responsibility you hold. For example, if you have a mentor, or even a mentee this is where you talk about it, briefly.

SECTION SIX: SKILLS & INTERESTS

Include IT skills (be clear about skills in Excel, PowerPoint and Word – they are essential for the workplace), your driver's licence if you have one, a first aid certificate, additional languages you may speak (even if you're not fluent).

Under your list of interests, remember that you are not looking for new friends, you're looking for a job, so they only want to know the wholesome, well-rounded hobbies you take part in such as sports (even cycling and going to the gym can count), theatre, cinema, reading books and listening to music.

SECTION SEVEN: REFERENCES

Contact your referees in advance to check that they are happy to provide a reference, send them your CV and give them some basic information about the job you have applied for. You don't need to give their details at this stage, just put "REFERENCES AVAILABLE ON REQUEST" at the bottom of your CV.

STYLE

When it comes to the style of a CV, we've seen it all – the good, the bad and the ugly! Here are some basic points you should consider if you want your CV to stand out in the right way:

FONT:
Use an easy-to-read, professional-looking font such as Arial, Times New Roman or Cambria in font size 10-12.

SUBHEADINGS:
Break up the information using subheadings and have clear divisions, but don't make your format too fussy by using lots of boxes or borders.

BULLET POINTS:
The information should be easy to skim read quickly so use bullet points instead of continuous sentences.

SPACING:
Add line breaks and spaces in between your subheadings so it's not too cramped.

CREATE YOUR OWN

Now that you understand what a CV should include and how this information should be presented, the next step is to work on creating your own. Turn over to see the Pure Potential template.

JOE BLOGGS

1 Education Street, Schoolton, UN1 1PP   joe.bloggs@unimail.com / 07123 456 789

EDUCATION

University of Anywhere   2:1 expected in Name Subject (BA)
St Whatever High School   3 A-Levels in Subject 1 (A), Subject 2 (B),
                          and Subject 3 (C), 10 GCSEs (1A*, 2As, 3Bs
                          and 4Cs including an A in both Mathematics and English)

WORK EXPERIENCE

Company & Co. – *Part-Time Marketing Assistant*   (January '15 – present)

- Organising…
- Consulting…
- Negotiating…
- Presenting…

Organisation Ltd. – *Events Assistant*   (June – July '14)

- Managed…
- Booked…
- Attended…
- Wrote…

Fashion Clothing Store – *Shop Assistant*   (Jan – March '14)

- Worked…
- Liaised…
- Assisted…
- Created…

PERSONAL DEVELOPMENT

Charitable Charity – *Volunteer*   (June – August '12)

- Helped…
- Ensured…
- Worked…
- Participated…

School Award for Excellence – *Silver Award*   (June '14)

- For excelling at…

OTHER

- Excellent knowledge of Microsoft Office
- Proficient in French and Spanish
- First Aid certificate holder
- Full, clean driving licence
- Hobbies include football, cycling and attending music festivals

REFERENCES AVAILABLE ON REQUEST

USING LINKEDIN

LinkedIn isn't just about creating your "online CV" and making work-related connections – it also has features and information that can help you choose the right course and right university for your future aspirations. These tools provide access to information about real graduates from these universities and courses, and insights into what jobs they have done on to do after university. There are over 450m people on LinkedIn and many have entered their education details, and then their subsequent career path, so the data is very robust.

Charles Hardy

Education Lead – *LinkedIn*

> **USEFUL RESOURCES**
>
> Download the LinkedIn App, or visit www.linkedin.com

EXPLORE UNIVERSITIES

Every university has a home on LinkedIn, and on that page (accessed via the main search bar) you can tap into the "Career Insights" feature. This tool pulls together information on thousands of graduates on LinkedIn who went to specific universities, and enables you to explore where they work and what they do.

Select a subject area and see where graduates from that course work. Select a company and see what courses are most likely to lead to a job there, and which are the top listed skills for people working there. In short, lots of information on real careers to help you make decisions about yours.

EXPLORE EMPLOYERS

Most companies have pages on LinkedIn. Use the main search bar to find ones you are interested in. Once on their page you can elect to "Follow" the organisation, meaning that you will receive their updates, news and job alerts into your own newsfeed. You can also explore the people who work there – what they do, how they have developed their careers to reach their current roles, what they say about working there. Companies often have included further information about careers and working there. Look for the "Careers" or "Life at...." sub-pages for cultural insights and employee testimonials.

Then of course there are jobs – either from the Company page or via the link in the top menu, you can search for the jobs you are interested in. When you view a job, you'll find more useful information on LinkedIn than anywhere else – not just the job description, but also information about the company, about people who are doing that job already, the top skills needed, and also similar jobs to that one you're looking at (maybe at companies you haven't heard of).

LinkedIn and these features are free to all registered users. Set up your professional profile (your online CV), including your work experience and educational qualifications, plus other awards and skills; add connections from your school / college / university, and your work experience; and get ahead with real insights on different careers, employers and jobs.

THE COVERING LETTER

You will usually be asked to send a one-page letter with your CV called the covering letter.

This is where you can discuss the skills and achievements most relevant to the position you are applying for in more detail. The covering letter, like your CV, is a very important document and could be the first thing a potential employer will read, so it must be unique to that company and impactful.

THE PLANNING & RESEARCH STAGE

A well thought-out letter is exactly what your future employer is looking for. Once you have spotted a vacancy which interests you, read the job description carefully and find out what they are looking for in their ideal candidate. Highlight which aspects of the job you feel, or know, you are capable of doing and the aspects that appeal to you, then look at the skills required and highlight which of those you have gained from past work experience or your education. You should have gone through a similar process when you updated your CV so keep your notes and use this as a starting point for this exercise.

STRUCTURE

INTRODUCTION

Start off by stating which position you are applying for, where you saw the vacancy and briefly explain your current circumstances i.e. 'I saw the role of Marketing Assistant advertised on GradJobs.com, and attach my CV for your consideration. I have just completed my A-Levels and will be starting university after a gap year…'.

HOW DO MY SKILLS AND PERSONAL ATTRIBUTES SUIT THIS ROLE?

Discuss how you became interested in the industry and support your points with examples of past work experience, knowledge you've gained from your course, or any extra-curricular activities which sparked your interest. Remember to reference any similar placements you've undertaken which will show the employer that you've got the relevant experience. If there were any skills mentioned in the job description that you have not yet developed, express a willingness to learn.

WHY HAVE I CHOSEN TO APPLY TO THIS PARTICULAR COMPANY?

Never, ever think a generic letter will do. It must be about the company you're applying to. Discuss aspects of the company that you find particularly interesting. This does not mean cut and paste information from the company website! Show that you have researched the firm and the sector - read newspapers (broadsheets, with business sections), company annual reports and research their competitors. You need to be able to say why you have been inspired by what the company has done and why you want to be a part of it.

SIGNING OFF

A weak, half-hearted ending to a covering letter can leave the employer wondering whether you even really want the job, so make sure you sound enthusiastic and super keen. The final paragraph should include a word of thanks, details of your availability, and how you're looking forward to hearing from them.

A. Student
1 Student Street
Megatown
City
X1 Z23
a.student@abc.com

20th July 2018

Mrs M Smith
Personnel Manager
Choice Supermarket
Any Road
Thistown
AB1 2CD

Dear Mrs Smith,

RE: Store Manager – Starting Sep 2018

I would like to apply for the role of Store Manager with Choice Supermarket that I saw advertised on GreatJobs.com. I am currently in my final year at King's College London studying Mathematics with Management and Finance, and will be available to start work from September.

Working with Customer Services, Merchandisers and Buyers during my summer placement with Big Department Store, I have developed an understanding of the role of Store Manager, and how crucial this position is to help the business become more efficient and profitable. I have also studied in-depth the most effective marketing strategies for fast moving consumer goods during my degree course, and I am keen to apply my experience to Choice Supermarket. Although I have yet to experience working at a supermarket specifically, I am a fast learner, and many of the skills I have developed will be useful for this role.

Choice Supermarket's market share has grown from 3% to 5% in the previous financial year, no doubt due in part to this year's brilliant advertising campaign. Targeting multiple market segments and highlighting the discounted prices of basic household products, and providing new niche goods and services has led to impressive growth, despite the economic downturn.

Choice Supermarket is an exciting place to work and I hope that the enthusiasm I can bring to the role, along with my relevant experience, make me a suitable candidate. I am available for interview for the next month, but will be on holiday between 8th-15th August. I look forward to the opportunity to discuss my application further.

Yours sincerely,

A. Student

A. Student

APPLICATION FORMS

For some companies the application form has replaced the traditional CV and covering letter because it is a standardised way for employers to collect key information from applicants without having to trawl through hundreds of CVs and covering letters in varying formats, lengths, font sizes and styles. Application forms work as a filtering process so employers can weed out unsuitable candidates before they go to the trouble of interviewing them. So, if you want to get through to the next stages, you need to put the time in and make sure your application form is up to scratch.

WHAT DO APPLICATIONS FORMS INCLUDE?

The application form will ask you to give much of the same information as on a CV such as your name, address, your school and university, grades and employment history. This information should be easy for you to complete, but just be sure to check and double-check all the details are correct before you submit as you'd be very surprised at how many students put down an incorrect email address or mobile number!

There will normally be a section that asks you about your previous and current roles. Make sure that you complete this fully, listing all of the achievements and experiences that you would on the 'Work Experience' section of a CV and making sure to tailor it specifically for the role you're applying for.

TIPS AND ADVICE

Have a copy of the job description to hand to look at when filling in an application form. Take every opportunity you can to link what you're saying back to what it says in the job description and try to use any key words you can see.

Read each question carefully to make sure that you're answering it correctly and to the highest standard. This is especially true if you're saying anywhere that you've got 'good attention to detail'. If a box isn't relevant, put 'N/A' (not applicable) in the space provided.

If it's an online form then draft your answer offline using Microsoft Word. This means you can do a spelling and grammar check. Save a hard copy and proofread the printed final version – its easier to spot errors this way, and will help you avoid accidentally submitting an incomplete application.

If you're filling in a physical form by hand, write as neatly as you can in black ink and practice your answers before writing them onto the form.

Get someone to read over your application before submission.

Finally, make sure you check the application deadline and get your form completed and submitted in plenty of time. You won't be able to give it your all if you're rushing hours before the cut off point, or worse still if you put your heart and soul into the application and miss it!

COMPETENCY-BASED QUESTIONS

Whether you're filling in an application form or sitting in a job interview, it is incredibly likely that at some point in the application process for a job you will be asked some questions along the lines of "describe a time when you have worked as part of a team" or "tell us about a time that you put your organisational skills to good use". Known as competency questions, these are often tricky to answer, but the STAR model can help you reply to the question fully.

STAR STANDS FOR SITUATION, TASKS, ACTION AND RESULT / RELEVANCE:

★ **SITUATION** - Open with a brief description of the situation and context of the story (who, what, where, when, how).

★ **TASK** - Explain the task you had to complete highlighting any specific challenges or constraints (e.g. deadlines, costs, other issues).

★ **ACTION** - Describe the specific actions that you took to complete the task. These should highlight desirable traits without needing to state them (initiative, intelligence, dedication, leadership, understanding, etc.).

★ **RESULT / RELEVANCE** - Close with the result of your efforts and include figures to quantify the result if possible. Furthermore, and perhaps most importantly, what new skills have you learnt from the experience that are relevant to the role you are applying for?

When using the STAR model be sure to concentrate most on the action taken and the result, and its relevance to the role you're applying for. See the pie chart below for a rough guide.

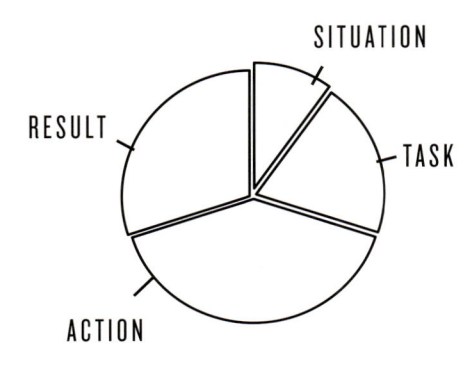

EXAMPLE QUESTIONS: WHAT IS YOUR GREATEST ACHIEVEMENT AND WHY?

The employer does not need to see that you've won an Olympic gold or found a solution to world peace, but a personal achievement that you can be proud of. If you have ever solved a problem, overcome a challenge or persevered with something then you're on the right track. What the employer definitely doesn't need to know is that you fluked something! They want to see an example that shows hard work paying off or difficult challenges faced rationally and logically – and above all a process or work ethic you can apply to future situations that can allow you to achieve even greater things.

DESCRIBE A SITUATION WHERE YOU WORKED IN A TEAM

Almost any job you can think of will involve teamwork. You will have to report to someone, or present your findings to colleagues, so make sure you show that you understand how important being a team player is to maximise performance.

The challenge with this question is that everyone, and we mean EVERYONE, has experience of working in a team in some shape or form, so it won't be enough to simply describe the situation. The way to stand out is to show what you took from those experiences. The employer will be interested to know what role you took within that team, and will be looking out for evidence of your ability to listen to, and be listened to, by others. Don't fall into the trap of thinking that the 'best' role to take in a team is leader – if everyone did that the workplace would be a nightmare, so be true to who you really are, and if you take a more passive role such as planning, executing, co-ordinating then talk about that, and how effective communication between all the team players is the most important thing.

You could also mention that, because of your age, you started by taking a backseat, but in future, once you've learnt the ropes, you hope to lead a team.

When choosing which anecdote to discuss think about any problems that arose, who tackled them, why and how? What observations have you made about teamwork going wrong? What about teamwork going right? Whether it was in your school sports team, a theatre production, academic project, or Duke of Edinburgh you should be able to find common themes, but make sure you talk about how this can apply to the job you want!

EXAMPLE QUESTIONS TO PRACTICE

1. How do you go about solving a problem?
2. Have you ever influenced someone to do something or changed their mind?
3. Tell me about a time when you failed to complete a task or project on time, despite intending to do so.

MOTIVATION OR STRENGTHS-BASED QUESTIONS

A newer line of interview questioning is focussed on your motivations and strengths. These questions look at what you enjoy doing and what you do well. Sometimes they will be asked at speed to prompt you to answer quickly (and interviewers hope more honestly!). These questions aren't asking why you're applying for the job or what your career goals are, they're asking what motivates you in life in general. What makes you tick? What gets you out of bed? You can find some examples of these type of questions:

```
What motivates you?
Which tasks do you get the most satisfaction from?
How would your manager motivate you?
What would you do in life if money was no concern?
What made you choose your current role?
Do you need other people around to stimulate you or are
              you self-motivated?
Do you enjoy working?
```

HOW TO PREPARE

It is very important to prepare for these questions so you don't respond with something that sounds unconsidered. Do some soul-searching - what is your motivation? We are all different, and we shouldn't be ashamed of being motivated by success. Examples of what might motivate you are:

- achieving results
- helping others
- team collaboration
- being rewarded
- performing in public
- thinking on your feet
- researching a topic in-depth
- discovering something new
- being creative
- travelling
- meeting new people and networking

The employer is looking for honesty here, so don't just say what you think they want to hear!

ASSESSMENT DAYS

Once you have applied for a job through a CV or application form, and maybe even after you've had a preliminary interview, you may be called to an assessment day. As the name suggests, they are a chance for the employer to assess your abilities through a range of activities, exercises and challenges. Examples of this include presentations, business challenges, team games and mock pitches.

PREPARATION

You may be given a rough outline of what's in store, or they may not give much away, so preparing for an assessment day can be difficult. The best thing you can do is research the company thoroughly - look at their website and their annual report for clues on their main revenue streams, their culture, and what sort of person they might be looking for.

As with any other important, potentially career-launching occasion, make sure you look the part, you're on time and you've had plenty of sleep the night before. The UK job market is more competitive than ever, so you need to give yourself every chance you can to show you've got what it takes.

TEAMWORK

Being friendly to your interviewers is a given, but what will make you stand out is if you are friendly, and even helpful to your fellow interviewees. Everyone loves a team player, so encourage and support as well as put your own ideas forward during the activities and challenges. It will show a level of maturity and leadership far beyond being bossy and getting everyone to do what you want.

If you feel you have let yourself down on one part of the day, don't be disheartened - you are being assessed on your performance throughout the day, so don't let your disappointment affect the next challenge, and approach it with fresh energy.

ENJOY IT

Finally, don't forget that everyone will be as nervous as you are. The best thing you can do is try to enjoy it, engage with everyone you meet, and ask plenty of questions - it shows you're truly interested in the role.

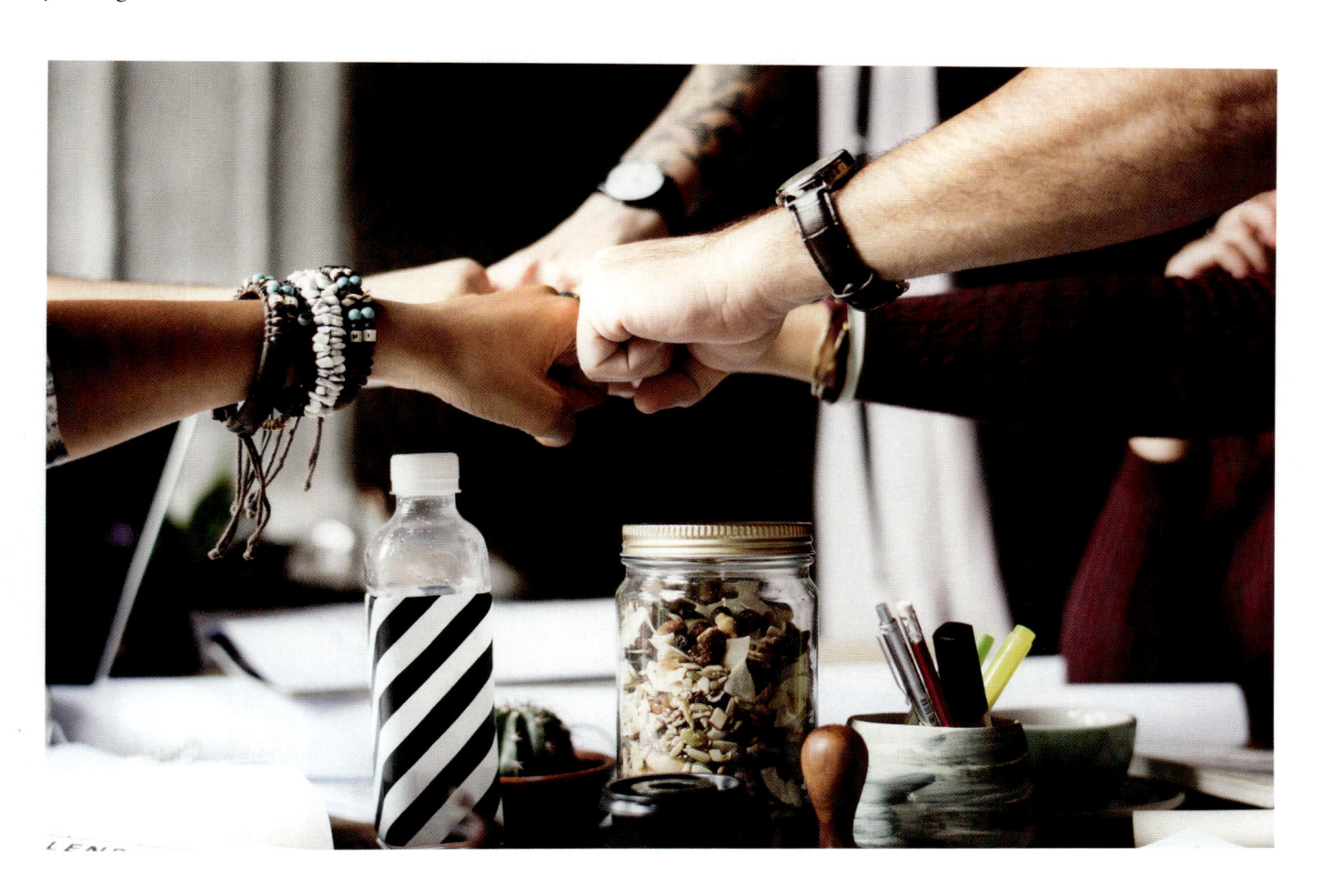

JOB INTERVIEWS

If an employer is impressed by your application, you may be asked for an interview. There are lots of different types of interview; the standard interview with members of staff from the potential employer, telephone interviews (which are just as important and some people find more difficult), video interviews (often via Skype) or panel interviews with several people grilling you. You may even get several kinds of interview with the same company as you progress through the application process. It's natural to feel nervous before an interview – in fact it would be impossible not to! Here are some simple tips on how to appear confident, and employable:

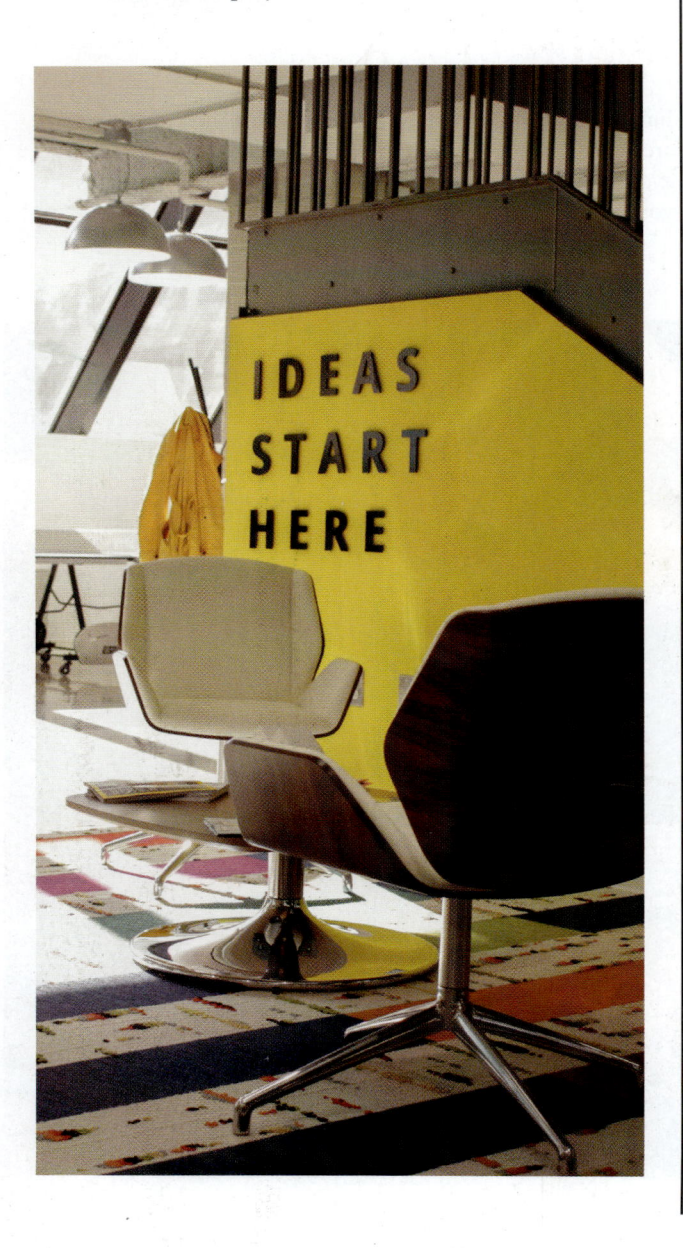

RESIST THE URGE TO FIDDLE

Don't play with your hair, nails, sleeves or jewellery. Instead use your hands to emphasise points.

DRESS TO IMPRESS

Try and find out the dress code of the office you're interviewing at. If in doubt wear a smart suit. Have neat and tidy hair, clean fingernails, make sure your clothes are stain-free and ironed, don't overdo your make-up, or wear shoes you can't walk in.

SMILE

Sounds easy, but when we are nervous we lose our ability to control even the most simple facial expressions. Make sure you keep your smile in check to look friendly and confident.

PLAN AHEAD

Plan your journey in advance so you know exactly where to go and how to get there, find out if there are any delays on public transport or road works on your route.

SMALL TALK

Don't be afraid of the old clichés about the weather or traffic, it's a great way to get started. Just allow the conversation to flow… and don't give a one-word answer to simple questions.

PREPARE AND READ UP

You should be fluent in the job description, the company and how you fit in.

SIT CONFIDENTLY

Shoulders back, legs to____ up, feet pointing straight____ in lap.

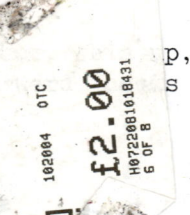